The CIVIL WAR

DIARIES & ARMY CONVALESCENCE SAGA *of* FARMBOY

EPHRAIM MINER

of the 142ND PENNSYLVANIA INFANTRY
and the 22ND VETERANS RESERVE CORPS

MARK A. MINER

Everett and Chris,

Thank you for all the
doors of discovery you've
opened for me.

Mark Miner

7/23/11

MCP

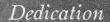

Dedication

To the memory of my great-great-grand-
uncle, Ephraim Miner, whose unselfish
suffering in the military service helped
preserve our divided nation during the
Civil War; to Thelma (Sanner) Gross
and her husband Charles, who lovingly
preserved his wartime diaries; and to
their daughter Kristi for graciously
allowing them to be brought to life and
publicly shared with everyone.

"We have seen them tried long and long by hopelessness, mismanagement, and by defeat; have seen the incredible slaughter toward or through which the armies (as at first Fredericksburg, and afterward at the Wilderness), still unhesitatingly obey'd orders to advance. We have seen them in trench, or crouching behind breastwork, or tramping in deep mud, or amid pouring rain or thick-falling snow, or under forced marches in hottest summer (as on the road to get to Gettysburg)—vast suffocating swarms, divisions, corps, with every single man so grimed and black with sweat and dust, his own mother would not have known him—his clothes all dirty, stained and torn, with sour, accumulated sweat for perfume—many a comrade, perhaps a brother, sun-struck, staggering out, dying, by the roadside, of exhaustion—yet the great bulk bearing steadily on, cheery enough, hollow-bellied from hunger, but sinewy with unconquerable resolution."

– Walt Whitman, *Democratic Vistas*

CONTENTS

Introduction

In the summer of 1974, when I had just become a teen-ager, and filled with curiosity, my parents took me to a Miner family reunion in Washington, Pennsylvania. I spent a lot of time looking at an old family photo album and asking questions. At dusk, as we prepared to leave, my great-aunt Jessie (Miner) Schultz walked to our car and handed me the album to keep. "You're the only one who asks me about these people," she said. "You're the eldest son of the eldest son of my eldest brother. And you carry on the Miner name. Now, go find out about these people someday."

Among many antique images in the album, one showed my great-great-grandfather, Andrew Jackson Miner, and his brother Ephraim and their wives. The photo is mounted

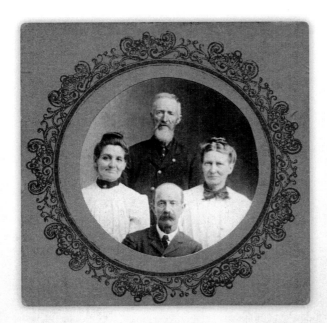

The photo that launched my journey—brothers Ephraim Miner (top) and Andrew Jackson Miner, with their wives Rosetta (left), and Mary Louise.

to a cardboard backing, and surrounded by bric-a-brac designs, portraying the couples in a studio setting. As Andrew died in 1921, I estimated the picture to be at least 50 years old; probably much more. He was bald and had a floppy, walrus-like mustache, while his brother Ephraim had a head of white hair in addition to a white mustache and beard. The look on their faces was stern. I knew that Andrew had lived in Washington, the town where our reunion was held, but the rest was a mystery.

Many were the afternoons when I came home from school and studied that picture—faces, posture, clothing—wishing I could have known them and asked about their lives. I daydreamed about their voices and what they would have been talking about as the shutter was being snapped. I asked several great-aunts uncles about the people in the photo, but they all had been very young when Andrew and his wife died, and didn't remember very much. The craving to learn about these relatives grew, but it wasn't until reading Alex Haley's *Roots* that I discovered how to start in such places as libraries with old census records, books and newspapers and in court-houses with deeds and other legal records.

After the death of my grandmother Monalea (Ullom) Miner in 1977, I found some old family papers in an oak box while cleaning out her root cellar. I learned that my ancestor Andrew was born in the farming village of Kingwood in Somerset County, Pennsylvania. My mother took me to the Carnegie Library of Pittsburgh, where we found census records showing that Ephraim lived in the Kingwood area as an old man.

The following summer, in August 1978, when I was 17, I took advantage of an opportunity to satisfy my curiosity. My brothers Scott and Eric were at a camp in Ligonier, not far from Kingwood. On a Sunday drive to pick them up, I persuaded my parents to take us on to Kingwood, to see what the countryside looked like, and perhaps to find some old graves of long-lost Miners.

My father agreed to my request, and after carefully checking a map, drove us to the very small town. Dad stopped the car at an old stone house to ask for advice on where to find cemeteries. Forrest Hall, the elderly owner of the house, came to the door and offered his help. I mentioned Uncle Ephraim's name, and Mr. Hall proceeded to smile, saying to my astonishment that he had known Ephraim, and that there were Miner relatives living nearby. He said that as a boy he had to shout loudly at Ephraim when talking because the old man's eardrums had been deafened by the roar of Civil War cannons.

Mr. Hall told us that Ephraim's daughter was still living, at age 86, in her father's farmhouse in a nearby hollow. He offered to ride with us to her place so that we might meet her. I could scarcely believe that an actual flesh and blood relative—and a Civil War veteran's daughter at that—was still living in 1978, and my imagination raced with excitement. We accepted the offer.

The route turned off the pavement down the steep, narrow dirt "Hexie Road," and led to a clearing with a barn on one side of the road and a two-story, green weather-boarded house on the other. After we parked, Mr. Hall led us to a side porch, and after calling to her through an open screen door, introduced us to a very tiny, delicate elderly lady named Minnie Gary. She was nearly blind and had been cooking jelly on her wood stove, despite

Meeting Ephraim's aged daughter Minnie Gary in the summer of 1978, on the porch of her home. That's me with all the hair, my brother Scott in the ballcap, and our guide Forrest Hall. [Photo by Odger "Wayne" Miner.]

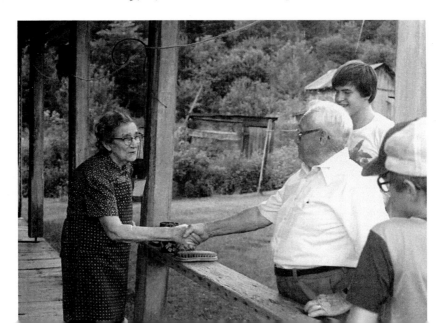

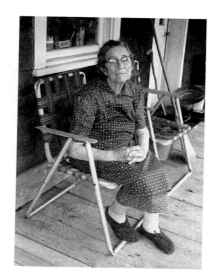

Minnie on the porch of her farm house in Somerset County, PA. [Photo by Odger "Wayne" Miner.]

the stifling hot August day. With typical forethought, my father had his camera in hand and began taking photographs.

I shook Minnie's hand and told her that my great-great-grandfather was Andrew J. Miner. "Uncle Andy!" she exclaimed. Without hesitation, she invited us inside, and we spent the next half-hour sitting in her kitchen, hearing stories about her father and his Civil War experiences, and of his brothers and sisters, all of them long dead. Although she could not see well, her mind was alive with sights and sounds of people she had known, including her beloved father, who was born 150 years earlier.

I told Minnie about my old photograph, and she smiled knowingly. She told us a story about one day when she was a young woman and was working outside in the garden, next to a small hillside. All of a sudden, pebbles and small rocks began to bounce down the hill in her direction. Puzzled, she glanced around but saw nothing, and went back to work. Soon after, pebbles and rocks again came tumbling down the hillside, and she took a second, more thorough look. She then heard some chuckles, and saw her "Uncle Andy"— my great, great grandfather—peeking over the crest of the hill. He and his wife Mary Louise had come for a visit, arriving unannounced, and stayed for several days. At one point they had a photograph taken together, and the two couples laughed and joked all the way to and from the studio. The picture that resulted, Minnie said, was the very one I had, with a nearly identical version hanging in her bedroom. It then dawned on me. The faces weren't stern, but instead holding back smiles, with one of the wives probably having just said, "Now c'mon guys, cut that out!"

It was at that precise moment that I first heard the voices of family history come alive, and my search for Uncle Ephraim began in earnest.

While I never saw Minnie again, I devoted much of my spare time over the ensuing decades to researching the life of her father, his siblings and their parents. I met many of Ephraim's grandchildren and great-grandchildren, in their homes and at family reunions, recording as many of their recollections as I could scribble on paper.

I learned that Ephraim obtained a government pension for his military service, that the National Archives houses original copies of all the pertinent paperwork he filled out to secure this, and that these files are open to the public. But I was dismayed to find that in a very rare occurrence, the Archives had transferred the files to the Veterans Administration in St. Louis, and were no longer accessible. In 1989, at my request, Pennsylvania Congressman Doug Walgren wrote to the Department of the Army's Reserve Personnel Center in St. Louis, asking for information. In a telephone conversation with a V.A. official in 1992, I was told that the files are "lost."

At some point in the mid-1990s, there were so many branches of the family that I decided to "shoot the moon" and find as many of them as I could, everywhere. The paradigm changed from tracing backward in time to exploring forward, from back in the long ago to today. As of this writing I know of the existence of nearly 2,000 of Ephraim's siblings, aunts, uncles and cousins, all born by the year 1900, descending in the genealogical tree from Ephraim's great-grandparents, Jacob and Maria (Nein) Minerd Sr., pioneer settlers of the Southwestern Pennsylvania mountains in 1791.

To my amazement, I discovered that there may well be 50,000 cousins alive today, and that the family surname has many variations, primarily Minerd, Minard, Miner and Minor. Another remarkable learning is that Ephraim was just one of more than 100 relatives (including spouses) to provide military service during the Civil War.

When the Internet was invented in the 1990s, I grasped that the new technology would be a perfect venue for publishing my research findings to share with everyone, and as a tool for attracting the interest of tens of thousands of distant, like-minded cousins, to broaden our collective knowledge and deepen our understanding. So in May

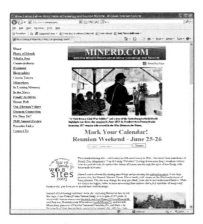

My award-winning genealogy website, minerd.com

2000, I launched the Minerd.com website, filled with biographical and feature pages loaded with names, key words and photographs, and with each bio linked to bios of parents and children for easy navigation. In 2003, it was named one of the top 10 family websites in the nation by a national genealogy magazine, *Family Tree*. Each Minerd-Minard-Miner-Minor soldier and relative mentioned in this book has a more detailed biography on the Minerd.com website.

As I wrote in *Pittsburgh Quarterly* in 2008, on the 250th anniversary of the founding of Pittsburgh, Minerd.com is intended to protect and preserve a fragmented family history and culture against the ravages of time and erosion of memory, public disinterest, destruction of interpersonal relationships and dispersion of families. When I too often hear of families breaking apart, I realize this website is an unprecedented way to re-connect everyone and to educate cousins and their families that regardless of where they live today, their ancient, unbreakable roots are here in the region.

In my search for Uncle Ephraim and the family at large, I have had the privilege of walking where he walked and viewing some of the very sights that he saw, on the battlefield and in the mountains of home. This rare experience has provided me with a profound appreciation for the self-sacrifice that he and his soldier-friends made for a country they barely knew when they enlisted but which they discovered in person during the fire and sweep of their wartime journeys.

Mark A. Miner
Beaver, PA
June 2011

Becoming a Man
1838 – 1862

Ephraim Miner was a God-fearing farm boy from a rural Southwestern Pennsylvania county whose life was profoundly changed by the Civil War. While briefly heroic in armed combat at the Battle of Fredericksburg, he primarily observed the conflict from afar, sidelined with injuries. He likely suffered significant emotional guilt as, enduring deafness, sore back and frostbitten feet, he sat out the rest of the war while many of his former regiment mates were wounded and killed in important battles—Chancellorsville, Gettysburg, The Wilderness and Petersburg.

Set into the broader sweep of Civil War history, Ephraim bore the first of his injuries as part of the Army of the Potomac's lone, brief breakthrough in what otherwise was a tragic, one-sided slaughter by the Army of Northern Virginia at Fredericksburg. He fought amid a who's who of military leadership, with Ambrose Burnside, George G. Meade and Joseph Hooker (Union) pitted against Robert E. Lee, James Longstreet, Thomas J. "Stonewall" Jackson, Jubal A. Early, A. P. Hill, John B. Hood and James E. B. "Jeb" Stuart (Confederate), names that all are deeply imbued in American military legend. Three times as many Union soldiers were killed at Fredericksburg than Confederates, but Ephraim fortunately survived. It is entirely possible that some of these generals actually laid eyes upon Ephraim for an instant or more, as he was among the massing blue tide of Union soldiers crossing

Ephraim Miner and his medal of the Grand Army of the Republic.

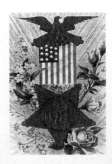

the Rappahannock River and assaulting the outskirts of Fredericksburg in the cold, foggy pre-Christmas days of December 11-15, 1862.

In later years, Ephraim told his children and grandchildren of the rivers of blood that ran at Gettysburg, which he did not see, because in fact he was not at that battle. Rather, he was in a military hospital in West Philadelphia. Of this he must have held terribly conflicted emotions. He shared that he had been so hungry that if he had seen a piece of meat lying in the mud, he gladly would have eaten it.

He regaled the grandchildren with another wartime tale about when for a number of frightening nights in a row, a guard of his camp was shot in the darkness every night. Each time, a large pig was seen grazing some distance away. In desperation, one frightened guard decided to shoot any living thing that came near. Sure enough, Ephraim recounted, the pig came around the next night, and promptly was shot dead. Upon examination, a Confederate's body was discovered under the camouflage of the pigskin. Tied to the tail was the gun he dragged and used to pick off the guards.

As an old man, Ephraim relished attending Civil War reunions, at which he and his colleagues were honored in high esteem, validating his service in the war, and making up psychologically for the significant time spent convalescing and serving out of harm's way during the conflict. At death, he left instructions that he be buried in his old uniform.

In addition to proudly serving in the Union Army, perhaps the most important effect of Ephraim's wartime experience was that he personally viewed the mighty country he loved and was defending, and made friends from all bounds of the northern United States. His wartime journey took him from the mountains of Somerset County to the battlefields of Virginia and to hospitals and posts in such cities as Philadelphia, Washington, D.C., Richmond, New York City, Albany, Columbus, Cincinnati, and Indianapolis. The back of his diary contains signatures of more than two dozen friends he made, fellow invalid soldiers from Indiana, Iowa, Maine, Michigan, New Hampshire, New York, Vermont and West Virginia. His eyes beheld the shattered bodies of friends, the not-yet-finished capitol building in the District of Columbia, large cities such as Philadelphia, Baltimore and New York, bustling navy yards and arsenals, camps filled with Confederate prisoners of war, hospitals teeming with wounded men in conditions of indescribable horror and the railroads linking the nation's major cities. Shunted from hospital to hospital, displaced by waves of new admissions of freshly mangled men from Chancellorsville and Gettysburg—for which the nation's medical community understandably was ill-prepared—Ephraim never settled in any one place for long.

While he does not mention it in the diaries, evidence hints that Ephraim had every opportunity to see a number of celebrities in person. Among them were Union commanders George B. McClellan, Burnside and Meade, wartime nurses Clara Barton, Louisa May Alcott and Walt Whitman, and possibly the commander in chief himself, Abraham Lincoln.

Thus Ephraim returned home to family and friends with an all-new knowledge that he was truly part of a nation, one he himself had helped to keep intact.

The Hexebarger valley near Kingwood, Somerset County, where Ephraim grew up and lived as an adult. [Author photo.]

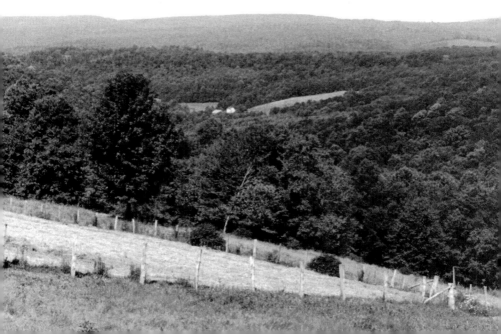

The diaries themselves are exceptional in their age and excellent preservation but not in revealing much depth of Ephraim's experience and heart. Perhaps reflecting his limited reading and writing skills, his quiet humble nature or perhaps a Christian aversion to braggadocio lest the Almighty disapprove, he chronicled his day to day story in snippets, as a log, but not as a record of the soul's journey.

To create this book, then, many other overlays were applied—a more comprehensive biography before and after the war, what was happening to his former regiment and the nation at large on the dates he writes about, as well as the wartime experiences of some of the more than 100 of his Minerd-Minard-Miner-Minor cousins who also served in the conflict.

After the war, everything Ephraim experienced for the rest of his life was through a completely different lens of perception. Returning to his familiar Somerset County mountains, in the quiet sheltered farming village of Kingwood, he slowly rebuilt his health and strength, married and had sons, lost his wife at a young age, remarried, had three more children, bought a farm and built a house, and struggled with offspring having significant mental disabilities. Deeply Christian, he imparted a love of faith and family to his progeny, and his example endures today in our national family reunions, founded by his great-grandchildren in 1986.

Early Life in Rural Somerset County

Ephraim was born on or about July 1, 1838 in a log cabin on a hillside near Kingwood, a sparsely populated region of Somerset County, Pennsylvania. He never knew the exact date of his birth, since the family Bible containing such details burned in a house fire when he was young. He grew up in a section locally known as "Hexebarger" ("Witch Mountain" in Pennsylvania German, a tongue in which he was fluent). His parents, Henry and Polly (Younkin) Minerd, were cousins, and he is believed to have been named for his maternal uncle Ephraim Younkin.

Ephraim twice married local cousins—Joanna Younkin (on his mother's side, from Paddytown) and Rosetta

Harbaugh (on his father's side, from Scullton). Although marriages of first cousins today are illegal in Pennsylvania, they were prized then, especially in rural communities where clusters of families lived of the same ethnic background and cultures. People of the 1800s had no knowledge of modern genetic research (which became a recognized science in the early 1900s), nor were there laws to prohibit intra-family unions. In fact, cousin marriages had value to ensure that like-minded couples with similar values and heritage stayed together.

As a boy, Ephraim attended some school and learned basic reading and writing, though his diaries later show an inability to spell consistently or to form anything more than basic sentences. Born with the surname Minerd, an Americanized version of Meinert or Meinhard, he used a variety of spellings such as Minard, Miner and Minor before later dropped the "d" altogether and settling on the simpler "Miner" spelling. In the decades before Social Security and the Internal Revenue Service forced Americans to spell their names with exact precision, it was not important for Ephraim to spell his name correctly.

Ephraim's lifelong place of worship, the Old Bethel Church of God in Hexebarger near Kingwood.

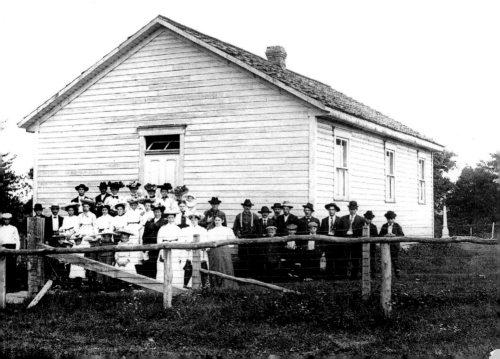

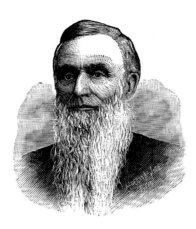

Rev. John Hickernell, a pioneer in the founding of the Church of God, including Old Bethel where Ephraim was a lifetime member. He later officiated at Ephraim's marriage to Rosetta Harbaugh. [*History of the Churches of God in the United States of North America,* 1914]

He was raised in a family compound of steeply sloped farmland, comprising about 500 acres which his grandfather Jacob Minerd Jr. had acquired in 1837. Ephraim's father Henry and uncles John, Jacob III and Charles each shared a quarter section of the farm, of about 125 acres each. On the Minerd side of the family, Ephraim knew 16 first cousins living on four adjacent farms within a radius of less than one mile, and another 36 first cousins living elsewhere, all born within a 46 year span from 1827 to 1873. He also had scores of Younkin cousins in the region from his mother's side.

Ephraim learned how to raise crops and livestock and raced horses through the fields with his brother Chance. He was an eyewitness to a triple tragedy involving his mother Polly, but miraculously may have helped to save her life. Tragically, she suffered from epilepsy. While holding a baby one day, she had a seizure and fell head-long into a lit fireplace, with her head, ear and hair badly burned, and the child killed. In one version of the story, Ephraim had the presence of mind to pull her out of the fire, saving her life. He later gave credit to God for giving him the strength. A grandmother, witnessing the horror, went running out to the fields to call for help, but fell over dead from the excitement. In another version, the grand-mother pulled Polly out of the fire, but died of fright after seeing the extent of her burns.

In the wake of this calamity, the older Minerd children likely were sent to live with nearby relatives while the mother fought to recover her health and the father strug-gled to keep his sanity. Ephraim likely was taken in by his maternal grandfather, John J. "Yankee John" Younkin. (The origin of the nickname is not known.) One day grand-father and grandson went hunting together for game. While Yankee John watched nearby on his horse, Ephraim lined up his target and pulled the trigger. The blast upset the horse, who threw his rider and bolted over a hill and was killed.

A second tragedy, a fire that destroyed the Minerd home, crippled Ephraim's father economically and rendered the family even more destitute. Why Henry was not assisted in rebuilding by his brothers on adjacent farms remains an enduring, troubling mystery. Sometime afterward, Henry sold their farm at a financial loss and moved to another smaller one a short distance away. By 1860, the year before the war erupted, Ephraim's parents and siblings moved to the northern panhandle of Virginia (later West Virginia). Within a year or two they crossed back into Pennsylvania, making a living as tenant farmers, a far cry from the role they once held as farm owners. Ephraim remained behind in Kingwood the entire time, in the care of relatives or friends, removing the father's burden to feed and clothe a strapping teenager.

At the age of 20 or 21, moved by the preaching and worship at the newly built Old Bethel Church of God, Ephraim committed his life to Jesus Christ, joined the church and dedicated his life to Christian principles. Old Bethel was built at a crossroads on a corner of the family compound of farms, and was the first Church of God planted in Somerset County. While the congregation had been in existence for several years, the site and building were not established until 1858, under the pastorship of elders John Plowman and John Hickernell. Ephraim is acknowledged in a history of the congregation as "an active member." Old Bethel, with its roots in the German Reformed Church, was a symbol of a national religious renewal among German-Americans in the 1830s and '40s, and was especially strong in Kingwood, where large revivals were held.

As the Civil War loomed with uncertainty on an invisible horizon, Ephraim reached his full manhood. He stood 5 feet, 10 inches tall, had dark eyes and dark hair, and a fair complexion. When the federal census was taken in 1860, he boarded in the home of farmers John and Elisabeth Dumbauld near Kingwood. They were near neighbors to Ephraim's 68-year-old widowed grandfather, Yankee John and maternal uncle and aunt, Andrew and Susan (Younkin) Schrock. The Schrocks later helped Ephraim manage his finances while away at war.

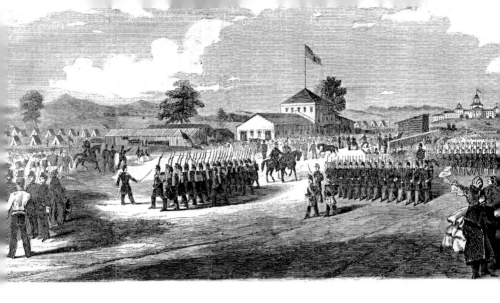

Civil War regiments drilling at Camp Curtin, Harrisburg, Pennsylvania.
[*Harper's Weekly*, May 11, 1861]

Outbreak of War

There is no record of how Ephraim reacted in April 1861 when he heard the news of the Confederate bombardment of Fort Sumter, and that his nation was at war. His response and activities for the next 15 months are unknown, during a critical period when the conflict escalated into far more of a mass slaughter than anyone could have imagined. While his brother Chance enlisted on September 19, 1861, just five months into the war, it was done over their father's strong objection. Thus Ephriam may have delayed enlistment thinking the war could not possibly last, or that victory was imminent, or fearing he would incur his father's disapproval, even when living many miles away.

On July 1, 1862, as the war's casualty count rose, and to fill the army's depleted ranks, President Lincoln issued a call for 300,000 new men. Less than three weeks later, on July 17, Lincoln signed a law authorizing states to begin a draft to raise these troops. Edwin R. Gearhart, who later served in Ephraim's regiment and penned his memoirs after the war, provided an insight into his own views which may reflect Ephraim's at the time. Writes Gearhart:

> *After this call I was uneasy, I felt I ought to enlist, why I did not immediately it is hard to say. Think it was a love of home and friends whom I did not like to leave and a little fear of consequences.... Ever since*

*I can remember I have always been afraid of some-
thing—cannon balls, especially.*

Lincoln's actions and the fear of the draft may have
spurred Ephraim and his friends into making decisions.
They may have preferred to control their own fate via voluntary enlistment, with the opportunity to serve with
each other and to remain together throughout. Or, they
may have been attracted by the immediate bounty payment
of $25 and a regular monthly salary. Two weeks after
the draft law was passed, when he was age 24, Ephraim
walked or rode the 25-mile distance to Stoystown, Somerset
County to join the United States Army. He was assigned
to the 142nd Pennsylvania Volunteer Infantry.

Also joining the 142nd Pennsylvania at Stoystown that
same day, August 1, 1862, were Ephraim's first cousin Martin Miner, whom he loved as a brother, a cousin by marriage,
Andrew Jackson Rose Sr. and a dear friend Gillian Miller.
From Stoystown, they traveled by train with fellow recruits to the state capitol city of Harrisburg to be mustered
into the regiment for a term of three years. This could
well have been Ephraim's first trip on a railroad line. After
arriving, they marched to the state capitol building, where
their eyes beheld the great dome they could have only
imagined before. After an overnight stay in the rotunda,
the regiment marched to nearby Camp Curtin to begin
basic drills.

Ephraim's enlistment immediately exposed him to a
wide variety of men and cultural backgrounds with which
he would have been very unfamiliar, given the insular
world in which he had been raised. According to George
R. Snowden, captain of the regiment:

> [They] *represented the diverse pursuits and composite
> character of the American citizen. Among them
> were the followers of the learned professions, men in
> business, bankers, mechanics of all kinds, drillers
> of oil-wells, miners of coal and iron, farmers, clerks,
> producers and manufacturers of lumber, teachers – in
> fact of almost every branch of industry – and generous
> and spirited boys from school, college, and the shop.
> The sturdy Pennsylvania Dutch were there, with their*

simple ways and honest hearts; the stern and resolute Scotch-Irish, the indomitable Welsh, the pertinacious English, the gallant and impetuous Irish, the steadfast Scotch, and the American of every extraction, Protestant and Catholic, all met on the same level of citizenship and patriotism.

In September, with only limited training, the 142nd Pennsylvania marched from Harrisburg to Washington, D.C., "arriving there just as the wounded were coming in from the second battle of Bull Run," reported one of the regiment's commanding officers, Horatio Nelson Warren, whose astute observations are reproduced throughout this book. "We learned from the wounded, who were flocking into the city, that the Army of the Potomac had been put to flight, and most severely handled..." For the second recent time the regiment saw a great dome, this time of the national capitol building. For a farmboy raised in the Western Pennsylvania mountains, the view for Ephraim must have been thrilling.

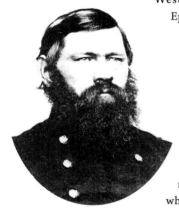

Col. Robert Cummins, commanding officer of the 142nd Pennsylvania, who was killed at Gettysburg [*History of Bedford and Somerset Counties,* 1906; Courtesy of the Carnegie Library of Pittsburgh.]

The 142nd Pennsylvania, led by Colonel Robert P. Cummins, was placed in the 1st Brigade, 3rd Division, 1st Corps of the Union Army, under the command of Colonel William Sinclair, Major General George G. Meade and Major General John F. Reynolds. Its first activity in Washington included guard duty and trench digging. "This was our first picket duty," Warren writes, "and, as yet, some of my men scarce-ly knew how to load a musket, and, while there may not have been an enemy within twenty miles, we could peer out into the darkness in our front and, in our imagination, see long lines of the enemy marching and counter-marching and getting ready to sweep us from the face of the earth."

They watched as other Union regiments marched out of Washington toward Maryland, to face Confederate forces at South Mountain and Antietam. Within the week, the 142nd Pennsylvania was ordered to Frederick, Maryland to provide care for the wounded of those battles. For the first time, these raw men observed "the horrible results of these battles," Warren writes, "as we saw them and heard of them from the mouths of those that were sent there, shattered and torn in every conceivable shape by bullets and shells..." While Ephraim was familiar with the blood and flesh from the slaughter of farm animals, he could not have been prepared for seeing the same brutal inflictions by Americans upon Americans.

In late October, the 142nd Pennsylvania marched to Antietam and Harper's Ferry to join the massing Army of the Potomac. Reports Warren, "This march was fraught with much that was trying to our experience, for, as yet, our men knew nothing about foraging, little about cooking and less about taking care of and dispensing their rations... In consequence of this, half of the time we were nearly starved."

Gen. George Meade, commander of Pennsylvania regiments during the battle of Fredericksburg.

The regiment was inspected at Warrenton, Virginia in early November by former Major General McClellan, just after President Lincoln had relieved him of command for ignoring orders to aggressively pursue the enemy. Ephraim and his mates stood in snow one inch deep, and as each one passed the popular former general, he said "Good bye boys, God bless you."

During one halt, at a camp aptly nicknamed Starvation Hollow, the hungry men of the 142nd Pennsylvania caught a glimpse of General Meade, the commanding officer of their division. As Meade rode by, they made loud catcalls at him for "crackers and hard-tack." Angered by such insubordination, Meade ordered the regiment to stand dressed in full gear for two hours in a rainstorm. After enduring their punishment, the men continued their march toward Fredericksburg.

The 142nd Pennsylvania arrived in late November at Aquia Creek, a military staging area about seven miles from Fredericksburg. They drilled for two hours each morning and two hours each afternoon and were under orders to march at any time.

Wintry rains drenched the soldiers and their tents, and many of the men became ill. Gearhart writes that while in the camp, the men cooked for themselves using a standard-issue tin cup and frying pan. "We were green soldiers and greener cooks," he writes, "and our stomachs that were somewhat civilized, often had to deal with a very barbarous mess. This, no doubt, was the cause of much of our sickness."

Cummins, senior commanding officer of the 142nd Pennsylvania, was stricken with fever at Aquia Creek and was unfit for duty. Alfred B. McCalmont was placed in temporary command as the deadly battle loomed ever closer.

PART II

First Action at Fredericksburg

On December 13, 1862, just two weeks before Christmas, the 142nd Pennsylvania faced its first battle-test of the war, at Fredericksburg, a refined, genteel town beside the Rappahannock River, precisely midway between Washington, D.C., and Richmond. Virginians held a deep reverence for Fredericksburg, as it was the sacred home of George Washington's mother Mary, navel hero John Paul Jones and President James Monroe.

Several excellent books are entirely devoted to the battle, among them *The Fredericksburg Campaign: Winter War on the Rappahannock* by Francis Augustín O'Reilly and *Fredericksburg! Fredericksburg!* by George C. Rable. Jeff Shaara's popular novel *Gods and Generals,* made into a film, features the battle prominently.

Expert commentators over the years have noted how brutally the Union was repulsed at Fredericksburg— Tony Horwitz's *Confederates in the Attic* calls it "one of the most lopsided slaughters of the War." Shelby Foote, in *The Civil War: A Narrative,* writes that "Of all these various battles and engagements, fought in all these various places, Fredericksburg ... was the largest–in numbers engaged, if not in bloodshed–as well as the grandest as a spectacle, in which respect it equaled, if indeed it did not outdo, any other major conflict of the war."

Thomas "Stonewall" Jackson [*The Civil War in America*]

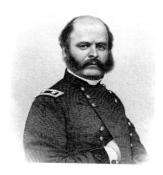

Ambrose Burnside, commanding officer of the Army of the Potomac, who led the disastrous strategy at Fredericksburg.

Warren, of the 142nd Pennsylvania, describes the importance of the battle:

[It was where] our first genuine experience of war commenced—here is where we passed the first ordeal that was calculated to try men's souls—here is where we heard the first rattle of musketry and knew and realized that the leaden missiles, screaming past our ears, coming directly from the muzzles of well-aimed muskets, in the hands of our common enemy, must deal death and destruction to our ranks, and summon many a good friend and comrade to lay his life upon the altar of his country and manfully meet his God.

Union commander Burnside, who recently had been tapped by President Lincoln to succeed McClellan, was eager to prove himself at Fredericksburg. He saw it as a logical place to cross the Rappahannock and press southward toward the Confederate capital city of Richmond. Under his plan, Union troops would cross the river on pontoon bridges and capture the town.

Unfortunately, delays in securing bridge-building materials cost Burnside valuable time. By the time his engineers began to erect the pontoons in early December, the enemy started shooting them from across the 440-foot-wide river. In short, Burnside's forces were heading

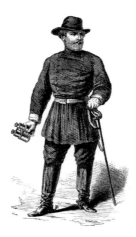
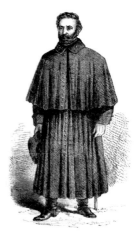

Confederate Generals Robert E. Lee, left, and Thomas "Stonewall" Jackson [*The Illustrated London News*, Feb. 14, 1863]

into a slaughter—a full river crossing and uphill assault in which more than 120,000 men were sitting ducks against highly trained, well-rested Confederate artillery. In *This Hallowed Ground*, author Bruce Catton writes "... the hills are just high enough to make an ideal defensive position.... In all the war no army moved up against a tougher position...."

Local residents, advised by Lee to evacuate, left their homes and traveled to safer places. Many later returned to find their residences destroyed or ransacked by Union foragers.

Ephraim and the 142nd Pennsylvania were not part of the army's assault on the town proper, but rather their attack took place several miles to the southeast, in what today is known as the Slaughter Pen Farm, a flat field leading to a wooded area bisected by railroad tracks. On the morning of December 10, Ephraim and his mates in camp near town were awakened by a drum roll at 4 a.m. and within an hour they were marching. In the cold morning air and anxiety of anticipation, the troops made as little noise as possible to prevent detection, avoiding their usual wisecracks and joking. Marching in the dark, they heard cannonfire toward their right, coming from Fredericksburg, knowing the ominous was at hand. Camping out in "still and frosty" night air, reports Gearhart, the men rose at dawn and took their place on a large flat field of land, but with great frustration proceeded no further that day. They eventually stacked their guns in nearby woods, and spent the night at that spot.

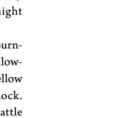

Confederate leaders at Fredericksburg: Jubal A. Early (top) and A.P. Hill. [Library of Congress]

While the 142nd Pennsylvania waited overnight, Burnside's engineers completed the pontoon bridges. The following morning, after the area was secured, Ephraim and fellow Pennsylvania regiments crossed over the Rappahannock. Gearhart writes about the stops and starts of the pre-battle activity of December 11 in great detail as the regiment stood on a bluff overlooking the river and the pontoons:

> *Here we had an unobstructed view of the flat lying between us and the river. This large flat was covered with a moving mass of "blue" flowing out over the*

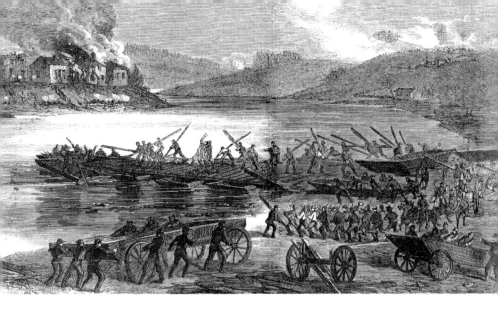

Sketch showing the Union infantry crossing the Rappahannock on pontoon bridges.
[*Harper's Weekly*, Dec. 27, 1862]

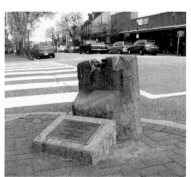

Old slave block, still standing in Fredericksburg, bearing mute testimony of its original purpose.
[Author photo.]

bridge, constantly and slowly something like molasses out of a jug. As soon as there was room, we descended to the flat. And as room was made, we kept getting closer to the bridge, but it was late in the afternoon before we reached the bridge and passed over. We loitered some upon the flat upon the south side and it was nearly night when we ascended the steep bank to the plain above…. Here we bivouacked for the night, building no fires. It was cold and the ground frozen.

Seven Assaults at Marye's Heights

The Fredericksburg battle that is better known today in America's popular culture took place at Marye's Heights, several miles away from the 142nd Pennsylvania, and is summarized here only for clarity and understanding, as Ephraim was not there.

After successfully completing their river crossing, following a heavy cannon bombardment and hand to hand fighting, troops under Major General Edwin V. Sumner occupied the town. It was impossible for the men in the immediate vicinity to miss a curious relic on the corner of Charles and William Streets—an upright block of sandstone, used not so long ago for displaying human chattel during slave auctions.

In control of the town early on December 12, Sumner and Hooker massed their troops and made plans to advance across a flat area leading up to the slope of Marye's Heights. There, heavily armed Confederate riflemen were perched in a sunken road behind a stone wall. The enemy's position was so strong that a Confederate artillerist boasted to his superior that "'A chicken can not live on that field when we open on it'."

The heavy fighting took place the next day, December 13. Most of the great written descriptions of the battle begin with the heavy morning fog. Pulitzer Prize winning author Douglas Southall

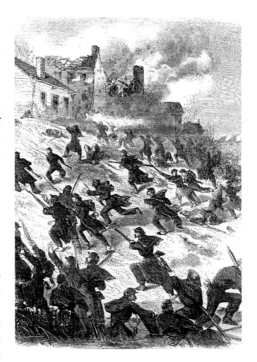

Sketches from Harper's Weekly showing the Union infantry crossing the Rappahannock on pontoon bridges. [*Harper's Weekly*, Dec. 27, 1862]

Freeman calls it a "swirling silver" while Catton describes "...a heavy wet fog along the river ... where no one could see three feet beyond the end of his nose." Gearhart writes that "A thick fog covered the plain."

As the fog began to lift around 10 a.m., on December 13, the first wave of Burnside's divisions began to march toward the heights. Writes Catton: "So the guns opened, and a tremendous cloud of smoke came rolling down ... to cover the river and the open plain and the tormented town, and presently tall columns of blacker smoke from burning buildings went up to the blue sky, and the waiting Federals saw walls and roofs collapse and bricks and timbers fly through the air, while men who had lived through Malvern Hill and Antietam said this was the most thunderous cannonade they had ever heard."

The first attack was repulsed, with a staggering number of Union casualties, shredded and maimed human forms scattered all about the slope. Another division moved ahead, determined to break through, with the same brutal

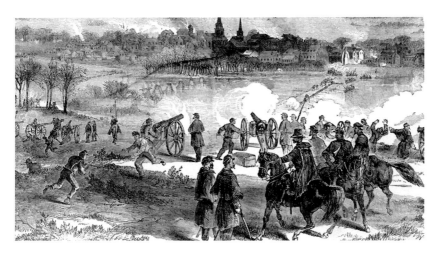

Union cannon bombardment at Fredericksburg. [*The Civil War in the United States*]

consequence, and a thickening carpet of bloodied blue-clan men writhing on the ground. Two more attempts followed, with the same devastating result. Shaken but undeterred, Burnside ordered more divisions to press the assault, facing certain oblivion but pushing ahead with an almost otherwordly bravery. One, two and three more times the Union infantry tried to assault the sunken wall. Each time the men were mowed down in a lethal hail of shells and miníe balls. In all, some 6,000 to 8,000 Union soldiers fell during the seven murderous charges.

Under enemy fire, Union troops begin their assault on the town of Fredericksburg. [From an original painting by Chappel.]

Viewing this carnage from afar, Lee was moved to utter his famed quotation: "It is well that war is so terrible—

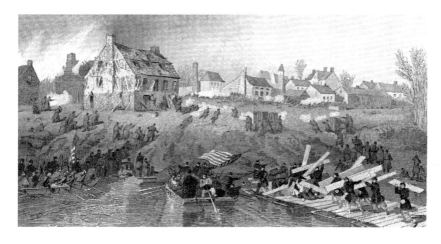

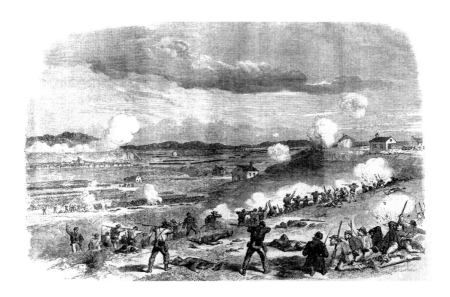

we should grow too fond of it!" Burnside watched in anguish as his divisions were obliterated, exclaiming "Oh, those men! Oh, those men!" That night, he told his aides he wanted to try again. They convinced him otherwise the next morning.

Confederates on Marye's Heights firing downhill at invading Union soldiers. [*Illustrated London News*, Jan. 21, 1863]

Ephraim in Action at the Slaughter Pen Farm

Several miles from the action at Marye's Heights, having crossed the Richmond Stage Road and taking their place on a large, flat cornfield known locally as the Pierson Tract, and later as the Slaughter Pen Farm, Ephraim and the 142nd Pennsylvania prepared for attack. They were part of a group of five Pennsylvania regiments—including the 3rd, 4th, 7th and 8th Pennsylvania Reserves—led by Meade. These soldiers advanced and soon made an unexpected breakthrough, the only one by the entire Union army that day at Fredericksburg, but were ill prepared for the force and terror of counterattack that was unleashed.

McCalmont, in temporary leadership of the 142nd Pennsylvania due to Cummins' illness, gave his troops a short motivational speech just before the battle began. He told them that "an accident had put him in command and he would do his duty and we should do ours.—'Let

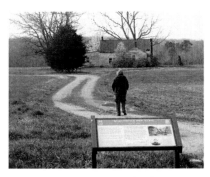

Visitor at the Slaughter Pen Farm at Fredericksburg today, walking in the same direction as Ephraim and the 142nd Pennsylvania, heading toward Stonewall Jackson's troops hidden in the far hillsides. [Author photo.]

the old regiments see that we are at least equal to any new regiment'," he said, as recounted in Gearhart's memoirs.

As the 142nd Pennsylvania began to march, they saw that "shells were flying over and around us, some bursting in the air, others striking the ground, tearing it up and scattering it around," writes Gearhart. "[The] cannon in front of us were sending out the shells, each discharge sounding like a heavy clap of thunder." The initial bombardment may well have shattered Ephraim's eardrums. But the record is scant on details.

The Pennsylvanians surged toward tracks of the Richmond, Fredericksburg & Potomac Railroad (today operated by CSX Railroad). They saw the first of the day's dreadful sights—"a horse hitched to a caisson shot in the head, several stretchers carried past with wounded, the blood dropping out upon the ground, a horse without a rider galloped past, his entrails hanging down out of his belly," Gearhart reports.

As they reached the tracks about 1 p.m., Ephraim and the 142nd Pennsylvania tried to press into a wooded area known as Prospect Hill, where Confederate troops led by Hill and Early, under Jackson's command, patiently laid low and waited for the moment of surprise.

Pushing forward, the left portion of the 142nd Pennsylvania met "good fortune" when they "stumbled" into a gap in Jackson's lines. Meade's Pennsylvanians had penetrated enemy lines in a place known as the "Boggy Wood" that Confederate officials had been thought impassable.

Near the tracks, the 142nd Pennsylvania began to unleash heavy fire upon surprised North Carolina units led by Brigadier Generals James H. Lane and James J. Archer. For a short time they "made great headway, crumpling up a couple of A. P. Hill's brigades, killing one of his brigadiers, taking prisoners, and just for a moment making it look as if Burnside's battle plan might make sense after all," writes Catton.

In *The Fredericksburg Campaign*, Francis Augustín O'Reilly notes that this singular place and time, when

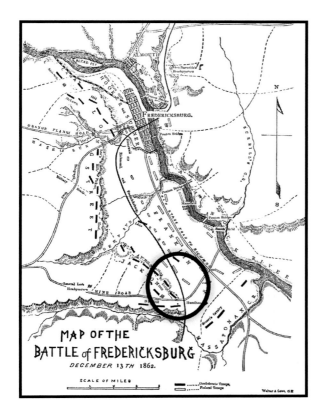

Battle map showing Meade's division (including the 142nd Pennsylvania) penetrating Confederate lines, as marked by a black oval. [Frank Leslie's *Scenes And Portraits of the Civil War*, 1894]

Meade's men briefly held the upper hand, was the "decisive aspect of the battle [which] pivoted on the closely contested fighting."

While the left hand portion of the 142nd Pennsylvania, including Ephraim's Company C, crossed the tracks amid the chaos, the right hand portion remained pinned there in a nearby ditch, firing as they were able. At one point the men were commanded to "Fix bayonets, forward, charge," and advanced to the tracks, but stopped, and continued shooting from prone positions.

Excessive confusion ensued. One Union officer ordered the 142nd Pennsylvania to stop firing, mistakenly believing fellow troops were in the way and thus would be under friendly fire. This forced the right of the 142nd Pennsylvania to remain halted indefinitely in the ditches along the rail line and to await further orders. Exposed

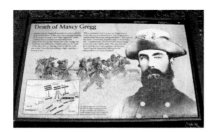
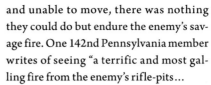

Tablet at the Fredericksburg National Military Park today, memorializing Confederate Brig. Gen. Maxcy Gregg, killed in the fight against the 142nd Pennsylvania. [Author photo.]

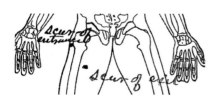

Actual surgeon's sketches showing wounds suffered at Fredericksburg by Michael A. Firestone (above) and Jacob Pritts. [National Archives].

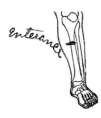

and unable to move, there was nothing they could do but endure the enemy's savage fire. One 142nd Pennsylvania member writes of seeing "a terrific and most galling fire from the enemy's rifle-pits…

Several of Ephraim's friends fell with wounds. Simon Pile took a bullet in the head, the ball deflecting into the roof of his mouth. Michael A. Firestone was shot through the hip and thigh and Jacob Pritts was hit in the shin, shattering his tibia bone. Among the members of Ephraim's Company C to be killed outright were David Ansell, Alex Hemminger, Harrison King and David Weimer. Horrifically wounded, William Nickler died two days later.

In this deadly hail of fire, the Pennsylvania regiments began to make a turning motion, with the 142nd as the pivot. They wheeled, with the 4th and 8th Pennsylvania toward the right, and the 3rd and 7th Pennsylvania to the left. They attempted to strike at disorganized units of a fallen Confederate officer, Brigadier General Maxcy Gregg, who was mortally shot in the spine.

But the maneuver failed, and rebel troops began a counter-surge. Frightened Union men began to run. The 142nd Pennsylvania was caught in a trampling of retreating troops, and abandoned its position. Writes Gearhart, "[The] balls were whizzing, shells bursting and men were yelling. I was making tracks at about the rate of three a second and I made them not very close together."

As they stumbled and sprinted in retreat, having tasted the terror of battle, Ephraim's comrades began to hear a most awful, intimidating sound for the first time in their lives—a guttural battle cry emanating from enemy lines—the "Rebel Yell." It was a high-pitched "woo-woo-woo" but described as hellish, spine-chilling, a regular wildcat screech, a yelping of banshees.

To cover the retreat, batteries of Union artillery blasted canister shot, firing until 8 p.m., well after the men had reached safety. It is possible that in the utter

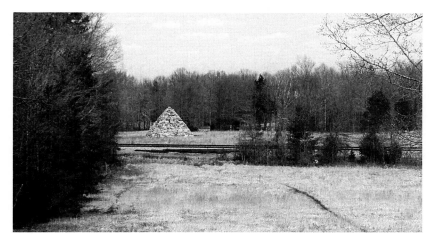

chaos of the withdrawal, Ephraim ran near one of these cannons, when it was about to be fired, shattering his eardrums during a blast he was not expecting.

On that patch of land, some 250 men of the Ephraim's regiment, representing one-third of the regiment's head-count at the start of the battle, lay dead or wounded. English historian George Francis Robert Henderson count-ed a total of 680 corpses, "lying in many places literally in heaps...." Snowden of the 142nd Pennsylvania writes: "The sacrifice was in vain, for although the division under Meade broke the hostile lines and threatened to turn their right flank, the only one which accomplished so much, not being supported by other and fresher troops within easy reach, the 142d slowly fell back, with a solid front opposed to the advancing foe."

Now safely out of range of enemy guns, the deeply shaken men of the 142nd Pennsylvania camped in a ravine. They remained there for a day and a half, awaiting orders.

As the men camped overnight, the weather turned colder. In a chilled wind and rain, a total of 12,600 Union killed and wounded lay across the wide swath of Fred-ericksburg soil, compared with Confederate casualties of more than 5,300. Sandburg writes that some of the wounded "lay forty-eight hours in the freezing cold before they were cared for. Some burned to death in long, dry grass set afire by cannon." Says Freeman, "The

90-foot-high "Meade Pyramid," built by the Richmond, Fredericksburg & Potomac Railroad in 1898 marking the federal breakthrough on the battlefield, and as a monument to Stonewall Jackson's headquarters. [Author photo.]

horror of the scene was far greater at close range than it had appeared from the lines." Another soldier observed that a Pennsylvania man, badly wounded in the leg, spent 50 hours on the field, after his "regiment had been compell'd to leave him to his fate." He was only rescued from the field under a flag of truce, after Longstreet sent Burnside a letter asking him to remove his corpses.

After 36 hours of inaction, as the enemy braced for new federal attacks, Burnside ordered his shivering troops to abandon Fredericksburg and to re-cross the river. Afraid the men would be shelled during retreat, pontoon bridges were covered in a carpet of grass and brush to deaden the noise of their marching. The night "brought a storm of sleet and driving rain, with a hard wind blowing eastward off the ridge and toward the river," writes Foote.

In his report to his superior officer, Major General Henry Halleck, Burnside defended his decision to draw away from Fredericksburg:

Battered Union troops retreating from Fredericksburg over the Rappahannock River pontoon bridges, two days after the battle. [*The Civil War in the United States*]

> *The Army of the Potomac was withdrawn to this side of the Rappahannock river because I felt fully convinced that the position in front could not be carried, and it was a military necessity either to attack the enemy or retire. A repulse would have been disastrous to us under existing circumstances. The*

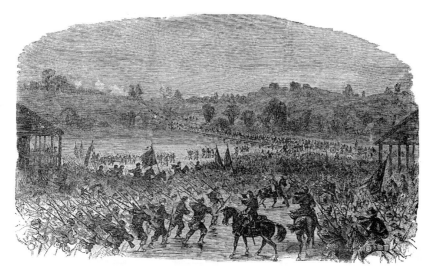

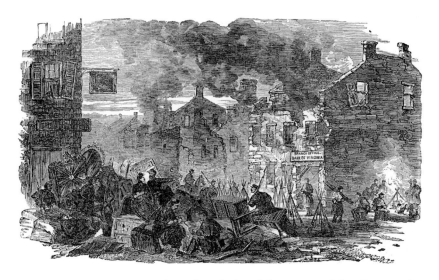

army was withdrawn at night, without the knowledge of the enemy, and without loss, either of property or men.

Ruins of homes and shops in the town of Fredericksburg. [*The Civil War in the United States*]

Shellshock and Fallback

Once their evacuation across the river was complete, the shellshocked men of the 142nd Pennsylvania camped in some woods about a mile and three quarters from the Rappahannock, trying to make sense of it all. Gearhart recalls seeing his regiment there:

...but how changed its appearance. Only a couple hundred men almost without tents or other equippage. The men were as dingy and muddy as turtles and the officers' uniforms had lost their shining qualities. Even the jokes of the wittiest seemed to stick to their lips and the laugh that now and then responded to them seemed like something "still born."

Despite his deafness, Ephraim was one of the more fortunate survivors, as he left the field without shedding blood, a fact which his grandchildren later pointed to with pride. One can only imagine his state of mind in the hours and days immediately following the battle. His eyes had witnessed the willful destruction of friends and fellow men, and he too had attempted to kill. His head and ears, throbbing under the shock of explosive cannonfire, could no longer make out sounds. His body, exhausted from fear, attacks and retreats, was forced to endure harsh wintry cold in the regiment's makeshift camp, likely protected at best by a canvas tent and thin blankets.

In this severe environment, his poorly protected feet froze, causing a terrible numbness and immobility. He could no longer hear, nor walk.

In summarizing their emotional anguish, Gearhart recalls that when they first prepared mount their attack, the men of the 142nd Pennsylvania were among a "well equipped and glittering host, 113,000 strong, every doubt was taken from the expectation of wintering in Richmond and celebrating the great event by 'hanging Jeff Davis on a sour apple tree'." But when that objective failed so disastrously, "The reaction was terrible, the gloom was deep...."

Battlefield Caregiver Angels

Having watched the battle from across the river, 40-year-old nurse Clara Barton tended to the Union wounded and dying. Better known later for founding the American Red Cross, she had served on the front lines for four months by the time of Fredericksburg. As she later writes, she was overwhelmed by the:

> ...hundreds of the worst wounded men I have ever seen... dead, starving and wounded, frozen to the ground. The wounded were brought to me, frozen, for days after, and our commissions and their supplies at Washington with no effective organization or power to go beyond! The wounded lay, uncared for, on the cold snow.

Her biographer, Percy Harold Epler, states that she "moved among them, and had the snow cleared away, finding famished, frozen, bent figures that once were men." While crossing the river to tend to wounded there, she was being assisted by a "kind hearted" officer when "a piece of an exploding shell passed through between us, just below our arms, carrying away a portion of both the skirts of his coat and my dress," she writes. Half an hour later, that same officer was brought to her—"dead"—much to her great sadness.

Poet Walt Whitman, who already had authored his *Leaves of Grass* book, but at the time was an unemployed news editor in Brooklyn, New York, fretted when he saw the name of his brother George on a published list of wounded. He traveled to Fredericksburg to find his sibling, arriving eight days after the carnage had ceased. Locating his brother who had endured but a scratch, Whitman walked among the wreckage of maimed bodies, feeling useless and help-less. He made a decision to stay. In a memoir, he later observes:

> The results of the late battle are exhibited every-where about here in thousands of cases. (hundreds die every day,) in the camp, brigade, and division hospitals. These are merely tents, and sometimes very poor ones, the wounded lying on the ground, lucky if their blankets are spread on layers of pine or hemlock twigs, or small leaves. No cots; seldom even a mattress. It is pretty cold. The ground is frozen hard, and there is occasional snow. I go from one case to another. I do not see that I do much good to these wounded and dying; but I cannot leave them.

Another battlefield nurse, novelist Louisa May Alcott (author of *Little Women*), helped nurse the wounded in a local house-turned-hospital: "All was hurry and confusion," she recalls in her best-selling memoir, *Hospital Sketches*:

> ...the hall was full of these wrecks of humanity, ... the walls were lined with rows of such as could sit, the floor covered with the more disabled, the steps and doorways filled with helpers and lookers on... The site of several stretchers, each with its legless, armless, or desperately wounded occupant, entering my ward, admonished me that I was there to work, not to wonder or weep; so I corked up my feelings, and returned to the path of duty...

Nurse Clara Barton, who tended to Union wounded at Fredericksburg, and who kept working despite a shell passing through her clothing. [*The Life of Clara Barton*]

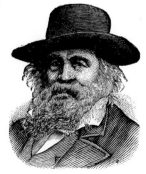

Poet Walt Whitman, who traveled from Brooklyn to nurse wounded soldiers at Fredericksburg. [*Local and National Poets of America*]

In their rounds, it is altogether possible that Alcott, Barton or Whitman laid eyes on Ephraim in the chaotic aftermath, or offered a caring hand.

National Aftershocks

The news of the battle spread quickly, producing despair in the northern states about the quality of military leadership and the waste of human lives. Front-page headlines printed in the days and weeks that followed. The outcome had serious aftershocks in the nation's collective psyche, especially in the investment community.

Historians J. G. Randall and David Herbert Donald report that "Sorrow caused by the death or mutilation of thousands of brave men turned into rage as the people wondered how so fine a fighting instrument as the Army of the Potomac had been used with such stupid futility."

The price of gold rose as the value of the dollar dropped to an all-time low.

The battle had such a scarring, profound and enduring emotional impact on Union soldiers that the following July, when mercilessly repelling Pickett's Charge at Gettysburg, they taunted their enemy with yells of "Fredericksburg! Fredericksburg!"

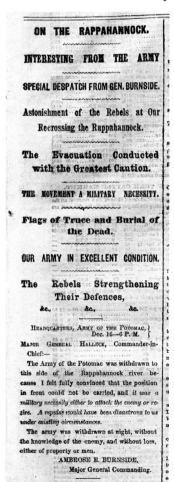

Front page headline in the *New York Herald* about the Fredericksburg battle and Union retreat. [Dec. 18, 1862]

PART III

Leaving the Regiment for Medical Care

Two days after their retreat across the Rappahannock, the men of the 142nd Pennsylvania were ordered to march a few miles to the Belle Plain Landing along the Potomac River, where they built temporary houses and chimneys to settle in for the time being.

Burnside decided to try to mount one more winter offensive and again cross the Rappahannock to make a final, all-out assault on the stone wall at the sunken road on Marye's Heights. He spent the month of January drawing up plans.

Cruelly bitter cold winter beset the 142nd Pennsylvania and other battle veterans in the days and weeks after Fredericksburg, undoubtedly causing Ephraim's badly frostbitten feet. [*Harper's Weekly*, Feb. 14, 1863]

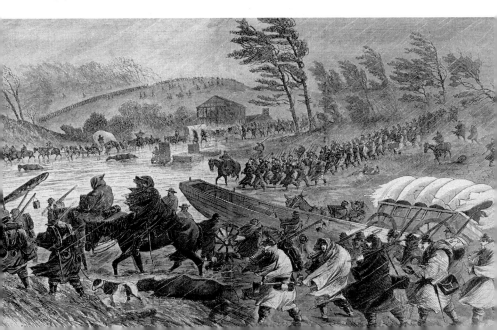

In anticipation of this new maneuver, Ephraim had few choices for treatment as the regiment's surgeons had higher priorities on their hands for what they likely concluded would be high casualties. On January 18, 1863, just 36 days after the battle, as Burnside prepared for his mid-winter attack, Ephraim's condition was more serious than doctors could manage. His loss of hearing left him unable to hear battle orders, and his lame feet certainly rendered him unable to march. He was sent away to a more suitable facility to receive specialized attention. His agonized thoughts or guilt at leaving his friends behind, after such a shared soul-searing experience, can never be known, but had to have been an awful, gut-gnawing ache of regret.

Two days after Ephraim left the regiment, Burnside's troops began to move. In a freak twist of nature, rare above-average temperatures and rains turned local roadways into mudpaths, and the army became stuck. Burnside finally countermanded his orders, which critics derided as his "Mud March" folly, and tendered his resignation. Lincoln replaced him with Hooker, and the army settled into winter quarters back at Belle Plain Landing.

The first leg of Ephraim's new saga was hospitalization at Windmill Point, along the Potomac River near Belle Plain. He did not remain there for very long, and the rest of journey took him far away from the 142nd Pennsylvania for the next two and half years, to cities and sites he may have only known abstractly from his limited education.

Treating his frostbitten feet was a top priority. While knowledge from his pension files is lost, clues do exist about the effects of frostbite on Ephraim's feet. One granddaughter recalled the significant pain he endured later in life, and that at times the skin turned black. A closer parallel may be drawn from comrade Aaron Zufall, of the 142nd Pennsylvania, also endured frozen feet "in the field" the same month as Ephraim, and Zufall's condition later was published in the monumental *Medical and Surgical History of the War of the Rebellion*. The book's entry on Zufall reports: "After undergoing treatment in field hospitals for several months, he was transferred to Washington and subsequently to Philadelphia. Acting Assistant Surgeon R. M. Girvin reported that at the time of the patient's admission to Satterlee Hospital, June 23d, his feet were swollen and purplish looking and he had not been able to wear his shoes for five months."

More than a decade later, when Zufall was examined again, the physician wrote: "The toes of both feet are stiff and the feet are very tender from the presence of chilblains [ulcers], which become very troublesome during the winter, when he is unable to wear shoes most of the time." When once more examined by a military surgeon in 1890, the physician noted Zufall's "loss of motion of the toes of both feet; cold and imperfect circulation. He states that the feet are numb and get cold easily. He cannot walk much." Ephraim's condition must have been virtually identical, lingering for the many decades of the remainder of his life.

Published analysis of Michael Zufall's frostbitten feet. [*Medical and Surgical History of the War of the Rebellion* and Carnegie Library of Pittsburgh]

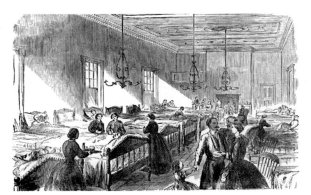

Military hospital in Washington, D.C., a scene Ephraim would have known well. [*The Civil War in the United States*]

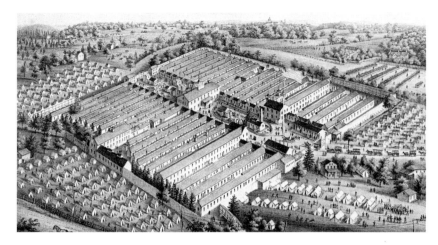

Bird's eye view of Satterlee U.S.A. General Hospital in West Philadelphia, where Ephraim was treated in 1863. [Courtesy of the Library Company of Philadelphia]

Hospitalized soldier being tended to by a caring nurse, labeled "Our Heroines." [*Harper's Weekly*, April 9, 1864]

From Windmill Point, Ephraim was sent in late January or early February 1863 to Finley U.S.A. General Hospital in Washington, D.C. He likely was transported there by rail, transferred to a government steamboat headed up the Potomac, and thence went by ambulance from the wharf to the hospital. Walt Whitman described Finley Hospital as a "little town, as you might suppose it, off there on the brow of a hill, is indeed a town, but of wounds, sickness and death."

Ephraim remained at Finley for about three months until about May, when, after a staggering number of wounded from Chancellorsville began to arrive, and doctors ran out of space, he was shipped to Satterlee U.S.A. General Hospital in West Philadelphia.

Encompassing 12.5 acres between 40th and 44th Streets, Satterlee was built for the express purpose of treating Union soldiers. Said one narrative, it was "perhaps the largest and most complete Army Hospital in the world." Some 35 medical officers served thousands of patients in 36 wards and an overflow space of hundreds of tents. Patients enjoyed a reading room, library and piano, as well as a sutler store, stationery and newspaper depot, barber shop and printing office.

At Satterlee, Ephraim undoubtedly experienced culture shock, given his Protestant religious upbringing, when he received medical and spiritual treatment from Roman Catholic caregivers. Among the hospital chaplains was priest Rev. Peter McGrane, while a dozen or more Sisters of Charity were volunteer nurses. An anonymous Sister wrote that in addition to Catholics, "Protestants were also attracted by the short but beautiful exhortations of Father McGrane, who said mass for

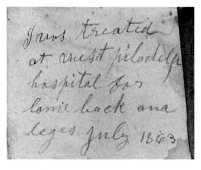

Ephraim's cryptic note in the back of his 1864 diary.

us three times in each week." Eager for spiritual content, and feeling homesick for his church back home, Ephraim likely attended these services.

After two months at Satterlee, in early July 1863, Ephraim and everyone there learned of the horrific fighting at Gettysburg, only a little more than 100 miles away. Satterlee received an immediate influx of 6,000 badly wounded soldiers, including members of the 142nd Pennsylvania Infantry. One can only imagine Ephraim's emotions as he had an unexpected reunion some with his unfortunate former mates. He learned that his cousin Andrew Jackson Rose was shot in the arm and likely would lose the limb, and that their former commanding officer Cummins was killed. A cryptic entry in the back of Ephraim's diary ruefully alludes that he was treated at Satterlee on the very days when his regiment was fighting at Gettysburg, something he was not willing to express directly or outright.

In this environment, Ephraim enjoyed the renewed companionship of his wounded old friends. One of them, Jerome B. Knable, makes this entry in his diary of August 1, 1863: "Saturday a verry warm day was at West Philadelphia Hospt seen Jacob Pritts Simon Pile & Michael

After the war, Satterlee was closed and dismantled, with row houses erected thereon. Today, the site is part of Clark Park. In 1916, a massive stone transported from Devil's Den at Gettysburg was embedded in the park as a permanent memorial to the hospital. [Russell David, 2011]

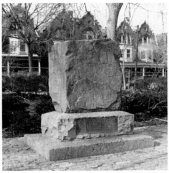

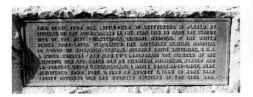

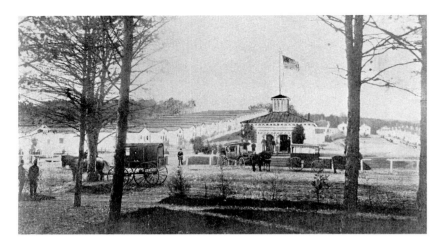

Camp Convalescent, Alexandria, Virginia. [*The American Civil War Book* and *Grant Album*, 1894]

Firestone & Eph Minerd." The diary also records day trips Knable made to Wissahickon, Manayunk and Philadelphia, outings Ephraim also may have taken.

Of these wounded men of the 142nd Pennsylvania, Knable was transferred to the Veterans Reserve Corps (VRC). Pritts, his left shin shattered by a minié ball, was treated in Washington and Philadelphia before deserting in October 1863, and later returning to Convalescent Camp, Alexandria, Virginia, after which he transferred to the VRC. Pile, a sergeant, wounded in the skull and mouth at Fredericksburg, was blinded in one eye, giving him a "very unsightly appearance" and giving off a putrid, offensive smell for the remaining 33 years of his life. Firestone, shot through the thigh at Fredericksburg, was treated in Washington and Philadelphia.

Later in August 1863, with Satterlee's headcount remaining high and physicians seeking every available bed, Ephraim was transferred to Lincoln U.S.A. General Hospital, one mile east of the United States Capitol in Washington, D.C. The facility was shaped like a "V," with two lines of 10 pavilions of housing. He remained there for several months, and at times stayed at Camp Convalescent in nearby Alexandria. (See diary entry for Feb. 8, 1864.)

Otherwise known as Camp Distribution or Camp Misery, Camp Convalescent was hastily constructed to prepare wounded soldiers to re-join their regiments. It housed 22,000 men who endured exceptionally squalid conditions. "Never anywhere was relief and sympathy more welcome or necessary [than at Convalescent]," said the United States Christian Commission, an organization created to provide religious and social services to the wounded. In reports, officials of the commission said this of the camp:

> *The suffering was unparalleled and appalling. Despondency and despair, aided by cold, hunger, filth, vermin, and disease, settled heavily upon thousands of hearts. Appeals to the Commission were urgent, earnest, terrible. The relief afforded through our delegates, though far from complete and universal, warmed many a poor shivering soldier, fed many a convalescent whose weak appetite rejected the hearty rations of well men, cheered with hope many a sinking heart, and saved many from the grave.*

Walt Whitman likely encountered Ephraim again during this time, as he made it his habit to visit all of the local hospitals, including Convalescent. At that camp, according to a Christian Commission report, volunteers "distributed wagon-loads of clothing, delicacies, and comforts for the sick; they have aided in securing hundreds of discharges for the disabled, written hundreds of letters for the helpless and the dying, buried many dead, distributed twenty thousand Testaments, hymn-books, and papers, and a million pages of tracts, opening and sustaining a daily prayer-meeting, and holding preaching services as frequently as opportunity offered."

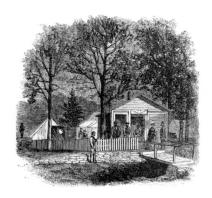

U.S. Sanitary Commission office at Camp Convalescent in Alexandria. [*Harper's Weekly*, Feb. 13, 1864]

As evidenced by his diary, Ephraim maintained contact with former regiment members during his recovery in Philadelphia and Alexandria, as well as family and friends back home. In the back of his diary, he tallied the number of letters received from mates such as Firestone (five), Pritts (five), David Gohn and others.

PART IV

The Diary
for 1864

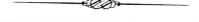

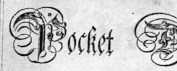

E Ephraim

DAILY

Pocket Diary

FOR THE YEAR

1864:

FOR THE

PURPOSE OF REGISTERING EVENTS OF PAST,
PRESENT, AND FUTURE OCCURRENCE.

CALCULATED FOR ONE YEAR,
BY SAMUEL H. WRIGHT.

New York:
PUBLISHED ANNUALLY
FOR THE TRADE.
1864.

[The first diary opens on New Year's Day 1864, with Ephraim writing at Camp Convalescent, Alexandria, Virginia. His words are shown as he wrote them, while the editor's commentary and interpretations are in italics. All of these entries and comments are in the present tense.]

~ January 1864 ~
Convalescent Camp, Alexandria, Virginia

Jan. 1, 1864 - I am well at present. it is very cold. it is new year to day.

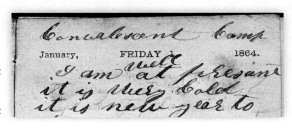

Jan. 2 - I am well at presant time. it is very cold.

Jan. 3 - I am well at presant time. it is very cold.

Jan. 4, 1864 - I am doing nothing to day. it is snowing. the snow is a bout to inches deep. I am well at present.

Jan. 5 - I am on gard today. it is cold and the snow is a bout fore *[four]* inch deep. I am well at present.

Jan. 6 - I am doing nothing to day. it is very cold. I am well at present.

Jan. 7, 1864 - I am on gard to day. it is very cold to day. the snow is about half a foot deep. I am well.

Jan. 8 - I am doing nothing to day. it is very cold. the snow is a bout half foot deep. I am well.

Jan. 9 - I am on gard to day. it is very cold. I am well at present.

Jan. 10, 1864 - I am doing nothing to day. I am well at presant time.

Jan. 11 - I am on gard to day. it is very cold and snow on the ground. I am well.

Jan. 12 - I am doing nothing to day. I am well. E E E *[Ephraim's handwriting practice of cursive E's].*

Jan. 13, 1864 - I am on gard to day. I am well at presant time. it is not cold today. it is cloudy.

January,   SATURDAY, 16,   1864.

I am on yard to day. it is a nise day. martin minarel went to the regiment this mourning I was soury that he had to go Camp Connalescent

Jan. 14 - I am on gard today. it is very warm but the snow stick pretty well. I am well.

Jan. 15 - I was in Washington to day. I nearley give out. I am well at present.

Jan. 16, 1864 - I am on gard today. it is a nise day. martin Minard went to the regiment this mourning. I was sorry that he had to go. [*Martin Minard, a.k.a. "Miner," was the son of John and Sarah (Ansell) Minerd. Ephraim and Martin grew up together and were less than two years apart in age. Both joined the army in August 1862, and were assigned to the 142nd Pennsylvania.*]

Jan. 17 - I am doing nothing to day. I am well at presant time.

Jan. 18 - I am doing nothing to day. it is raining to day. I am well this day. one year ago I left the regiment. [*Ephraim refers to his transfer from a field hospital to Windmill Point for treatment after the Battle of Fredericksburg, and just before the aborted "Mud March."*]

Jan. 19, 1864 - I am on gard to day. it is very mudy. I am well at present.

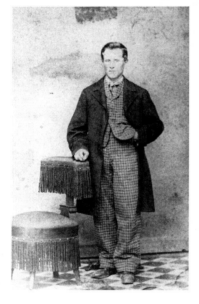

Martin Miner, Ephraim's cousin and fellow member of the 142nd Pennsylvania.

Jan. 20 - I am doing nothing only I washed today. I am well at presant time. the snow is all gone a way but it is very cold.

Jan. 21 - I am on gard today. I am well at present.

Jan. 22, 1864 - I am doing nothing to day only out on the inspection of armes.

Jan. 23 - I am doing nothing to day. I am well at presant time. it is a very nise day.

Jan. 24 - I am on gard to day. I am well at presant time. it is a nise day very plesant.

Jan. 25, 1864 - I am doing nothing to day. am well at presant time. it is a very nise day very warm.

Jan. 26 - I am on gard to day. it is a very nise day. it is very warm. I am well at presant time.

Jan. 27 - I was in Washington to day. we took som inverlids [*invalids*] to Washington. I nearly give out.

Jan. 28, 1864 - I just got back from Washington. it is twelve oclock.

Jan. 29 - I was in Washington to day. I nearly give out. I am well.

Jan. 30 - I just got back from Washington.

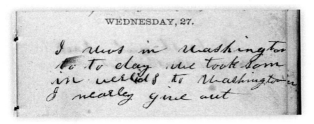

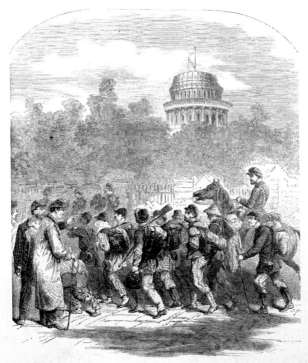

Convalescent soldiers marching near the unfinished dome of the capitol building in Washington. D.C. [*Harper's Weekly*, Nov. 15, 1862]

Jan. 31, 1864 - I am doing nothing today. I am well at present.

~ February 1864 ~

Feb. 1, 1864 - I am on gard to day. it is raining to day. I am well at presant time.

Feb. 2 - I am doing nothing to day. I am well at presant. it is very mudy to day. *[Far away from Ephraim, Captain Horatio Warren is promoted to Major of the 142nd Pennsylvania, and later is elevated to colonel at the Battle of Five Forks.]*

Feb. 3, 1864 - I am doing nothing to day. I am well at presant. it is very cold to day.

Feb. 4 - I am on gard to day. it is very cold. I am well at present.

Feb. 5 - I am doing nothing to day. I am well at presant. it is a very nise day.

Feb. 6, 1864 - I am on gard to day. I am well at presant. it is cloudy. it looks for raine. it is very warm. *[The 142nd Pennsylvania is involved on the Rapidan on February 6 - 7, 1864, and then is on duty at Culpeper until May 1864.]*

Feb. 7 - I am doing nothing to day. I was on camand. I am market for the hospital.

Feb. 8 - This mourning I left Convalescent Camp and went to lincoln hospital.

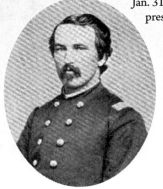

Horatio Nelson Warren, commanding one of the commanding officers of the 142nd Pennsylvania. His writings offer insights into the regiment's activities.
[War History]

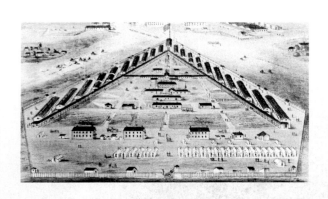

Lincoln Hospital, a mile from the nation's capitol, where Ephraim convalesced in the winter of 1864. [Sanders & Company, 1865]

Feb. 9, 1864 - I was axamend [examined] this mourning. we was sent back to Convalescent Camp and then tha [they] sent us right back again to lincoln hospital a gaine.

Feb. 10 - Wm H. Price, Co. B 110 Pa vols, Washington DC [Signature]

WEDNESDAY, 10.

Feb. 11 - F. Iams, co D 140 P V, Washington DC, care of louiten van dyke [Signature. Franklin F. Iams stands 5 feet, 9½ inches tall and is a teacher before the war. He serves in the 140th Pennsylvania Infantry with Ephraim's future nephew by marriage, Cyrus Lindley, and cousin Henry "Foxy" McKnight. At Petersburg in 1864, he is shot in the leg, with the ball fracturing the fibula and exiting through the calf. He is recommended for transfer to the Veterans Reserve Corps (VRC), but is found unfit, so is discharged at Carver Hospital in Washington, D.C. in 1865. He marries Mary E. Bane and has two children: George L. and Mary F. Iams. Physicians examining Iams in the 1880s note impaired walking and ankle motion. He dies at age 69 on May 3, 1906, and is buried in Amity.]

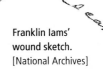

Franklin Iams' wound sketch.
[National Archives]

Lincoln Hospital

[Walt Whitman spends many months visiting the wounded in Washington, including at Convalescent Camp and Lincoln Hospital, where he likely sees Ephraim. He writes of "washing and dressing wounds," as well as providing the "poor chaps" with pencils and papers, inexpensive pocket diaries and almanacs, as well as newspapers and magazines. Ephraim's diary could well have been a gift directly from Whitman. "In camp and everywhere, I was in the habit of reading or giving recitations to the men," Whitman writes. "They were very fond of it... We would gather in a large group by ourselves, after supper, and spend the time in such readings, or in talking, and occasionally by an amusing game called the game of twenty questions."]

Feb. 12, 1864 - to day I got back to lincoln hospital. Ephraim Minard. [signs his name in cursive script]

Feb. 13 - I am not well to day. it is very cold.

Feb. 14 - I am little beter to day. it is very winday and cold.

Feb. 15, 1864 - I am a little beter to day. it is snowing this after noon. it is very cold.

Feb. 16 - I am most well. the snow is to inch deep but is nearly all gone a way. the sun shines but it is very winday.

Feb. 17 - I am well at presant time. it is very cold and windy.

Feb. 18, 1864 - I am well at presant. it is heape warmer to day then what it was yesteday. the sun shines very warm.

Feb. 19 - I am well at presant. it is very cold to day but the sun shines very brite and clear but it is very cold.

Feb. 20 - I am well at presant time. I was in Washington to day. I had a good time. I was down in the navy yard to day and I seen graite maney [great many] works. it is a nise day. [The yard is a major ordnance manufacturing and ship repair facility, and of strategic importance in the defense of Washington, D.C.]

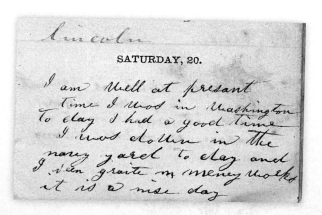

WELL AT THIS TIME

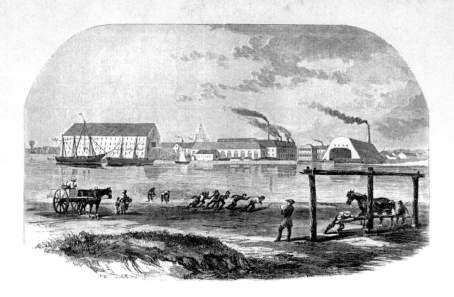

Feb. 21, 1864 - I am well at presant time. it is a very nise day to day.

Washington Navy Yard.
[*Harper's Weekly*,
April 20, 1861]

Feb. 22 - I am well at presant time. it is a nise day. I am stil at lincoln hospital.

Feb. 23 - I am well at presant time. the wether is very nise. it is all most warm. is in the spring.

Feb. 24, 1864 - I am well at presant time. it is very nise wether. I am at work. I am white washing the wardes.

Feb. 25 - I am well at presant. it is a very nise day.

Feb. 26 - I am well at presant time. it is a very nise day today.

Feb. 27, 1864 - I am well at presant time. it is a very nise day. I am abote ready to get to the city of Washington. it is five oclock now. [*The first Union prisoners begin to arrive at the notorious Andersonville prison camp in Camp Sumter, South Carolina. By the end of summer, Andersonville holds 33,000 POWs.*]

Feb. 28 - I am well at presant time. it is a very nise day.

Feb. 29 - I am well at presant time. it is cloudy to day. it look for snow. it is cold. the last day of febury.

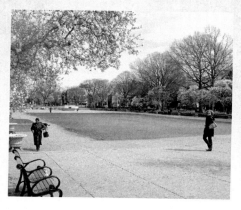
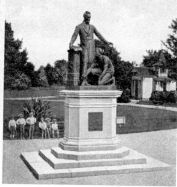

Left: Lincoln Park, Washington D.C., site of the former Lincoln Hospital where Ephraim convalesced and where poet Walt Whitman nursed wounded soldiers. [Author photo.]

Right: Lincoln Emancipation Statue, also known as the Freedom's Memorial, erected 1876 at the former site of Lincoln Hospital.

~ *March 1864* ~

March 1, 1864 - I am not well at presant. I feel bad. my bownes paines wery *[bones pain weary]*. it snowed last knight. the snow is a bout to inches deep. it is raining to day.

March 2 - I am well at presant time. it is a nise day to day. the snow is going away. it is mudy.

March 3 - I am well at presant time. it is a very nise day.

March 4, 1864 - I am well at present time. it is a very nise day. I am white washing to day.

March 5 - I am well at presant time. it is raining to day. I am doing nothing to day. it is not cold.

March 6 - I am well at presant time. it is cold to day and winday.

March 7, 1864 - I am well at presant time. I am white washing to day. it is cold.

March 8 - I am well at presant time. I am doing nothing do day. it is raining to day.

March 9 - I am well at presant time. it is a very nise day. *[Dissatisfied with the under-performance of his generals, President Lincoln appoints Ulysses S. Grant as lieutenant general in command of all United States Army forces.]*

March 10, 1864 - I am well at presant time. it is raining to day. it is a cold rain.

March 11 - I am well at presant time. it is raining to day. very cold rain.

March 12 - I am well at presant time. I am white washing to day. I am going to town to night. it is very nise day.

March 13, 1864 - I am well at presant time. I was in town last knight.

I was in a candobery [Canterbury]. thare was very good performance. there was six girles came out on the flore and danced. I never seen beter dancing. [The Canterbury music hall on Louisiana Avenue is a popular entertainment spot for soldiers in Washington. In April 1865, John Wilkes Booth and his co-conspirators Samuel Arnold, George Atzerodt, Michael O'Laughlin and Mary Surratt meet at Canterbury to initially plan what is to be President Lincoln's kidnapping. The night before Booth shoots Lincoln, O'Laughlin makes a stop at Canterbury before backing out of the plot when he learns that the true purpose is to assassinate the president and his cabinet.]

March 14 - I am well at presant time. I am white washing to day. it is a very nice day.

March 15 - I am well at presant time. I am white washing. it is cold to day.

March 16, 1864 - I am well at presant time. I am doing nothing today. it is very cold.

March 17 - I am well at presant time. it is very cold to day. [Ephraim's cousin Albert Miner, of the 19th Ohio Infantry, dies in captivity as a prisoner in a Confederate hospital in Danville, Virginia.]

March 18 - I am well at presant time. I cind [signed] the pay roles to day.

March 19, 1864 - I am well at presant time. I was working this fournoon.

March 20 - I am well at presant time. it is a nice day. I am a going to tak walk this afternoon down to the river.

March 21 - I am well at presant time. I am white washing to day. it is cold. I am going to town to knight.

March 22, 1864 - I am well at the presant time. I am doing nothing to day. it is ofel cold and windy. it is a going to snow. I am going to town to knight.

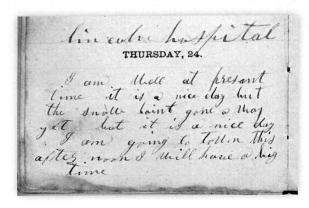

March 23 - I am well at presant time. I am doing nothing to day. the snow is a bout foot deep this mourning. it is ofel cold.

March 24 - I am well at presant time. it is a nice day but the snow haint gone a way yet but it is a nice day I am going to town this afternoon. I will have a big time. [*Note Ephraim's use of the colloquial "hain't" for "has not."*]

March 25, 1864 - I am well at presant. it is very cold. it raind very hard last knigt.

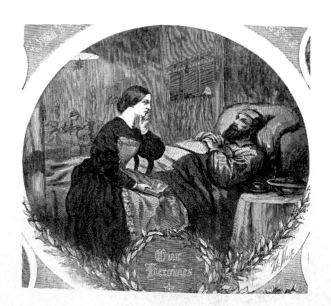

Newspaper engraving of a Union hospital scene. [*Harper's Weekly*, April 9, 1864]

March 26 - I am well at presant. I am going to town this evening.

March 27 - I am not well to day. I feel very bad at presant. it is a very nice day.

March 31, 1864 - I am not well this mourning. it is cold the last day of March.

~ April 1864 ~

April 1 - I am well at presant time. I am white washing. I am going in the city this after noon. it is raining.

April 2 - I am well at presant. I am doing nothing to day. it is snowing and som rain. it is very bad day.

April 3, 1864 - I am well at presant. I am very lonesom to day. I am all ways lone som on Sundays.

April 4 - I am well at presant. I white washing today. it is raining this after noon. I am going to town this eavening.

April 5 - I am well at presant time. it is raining to day. it is a cold raine.

April 6, 1864 - I am well at presant time. it is cold.

April 7 - I am well at presant time.

April 8 - I am well at presant time. it is a very nice day. [Ephraim's cousin by marriage, Sylvester Georgia (husband of Laveria Minerd), of the 28th Iowa Infantry, is captured near Mansfield, Louisiana.]

April 9, 1864 - I am well at presant time. it is raining to day. it is a very cold raine. I am white washing to day.

April 10 - I am well at presant time. it is cloudy to day. it is very mudy.

April 11 - I am well at presant. it is a very nice day. I am white washing.

April 12, 1864 - I am well at presant. it is a nice day. I am white washing.

April 13 - I am well at presant. it is a beautifull day. I am white washing.

April 14 - I am not well to day. it is a very nice day. I am white washing.

April 15, 1864 - I am no beter to day. I feel very bad. I cant work to day for I am to sick.

April 16 - I am well at presant time. it a nice day.

April 17 - I am well at presant. it is a nice day.

April 18, 1864 - I am well at presant time. it is a nice day to day.

April 19 - I am well at presant time.

April 20 - I am well at presant. it is a very nice day.

April 21, 1864 - I am well at presant. it is a very nice day. I am working at the white washing.

April 22 - I am well at presant. it is a beautiful day.

April 23 - I am well at presant. it is a nice day.

April 24, 1864 - I am well a presant time. it is a very nice day.

April 25 - I am well at presant time. it is a very nice day.

April 26 - I am well at presant time. it is a nice day very plesant.

April 27, 1864 - I am well at presant time. it is very windy to day.

April 28 - I am well at presant time. it is very cold this mourning.

April 29 - I am well at presant time. it is a very nice day.

April 30, 1864 - I am well at presant time. it is very nice day to day. I was musterd to day the last day of April.

lincoln hospital

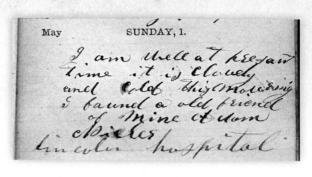

May 1, 1864 - I am well at presant time. it is cloudy and cold this mourning. I found a old friend of mine Adam Nicles [*Adam Nickelson is in the 142nd Pennsylvania. Suffering from a lingering bad cold, and sore legs and breast, he is treated at Culpeper, Virginia, and then sent to Lincoln Hospital. He later is transferred to a hospital on Narragansett Bay in Rhode Island. After the war, he lives in and around Confluence, Somerset County, and marries Rosetta Eicher (who died in childbirth the year after marriage) and Maria Snyder. His children are William L., Edward B., Levi E., Sarah E., Susan H., James G., Jacob A., Silas A. and Annie May Nickelson. In August 1924, he attends the 1924 Minerd-Miner Reunion at Confluence. He dies of hardening of the arteries on Christmas Day 1934, at the age of 94.*]

May 2 - I am well at presant time. it is cold to day and windy.

May 3, 1864 - I am well at presant time. I am going to the city to knight.

May 4 - I am well at presant time. I was down in the city last knight. I had a good time.

Battle of the Wilderness, May 5, 1864, in which the 142nd Pennsylvania was engaged in action.

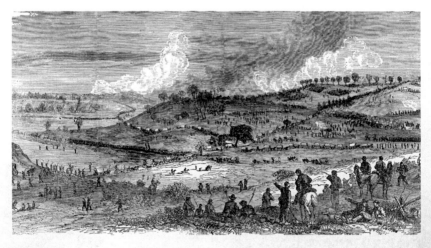

May 5 - I am well at presant time. *[The 142ⁿᵈ Pennsylvania is engaged in the Battles of the Wilderness, pitting Grant and Meade again versus Lee. Nearly 163,000 troops fight to an inconclusive result in dense woods along the Orange Turnpike and Plank Road. Estimated casualties: 29,800.]*

May 6, 1864 - I am well at presant time. it is very nice wether very warm. I was in town last knight. I had a good time.

May 7 - I am well at presant time. it is very hot and dri.

May 8 - I am well at presant time. it is very hot and dri. *[The 142ⁿᵈ Pennsylvania sees action at Laurel Hill and then at Spotsylvania Court House during a five-day period. During this battle, Union forces under Grant and Meade march toward Richmond, but meet resistance at Spotsylvania. Warren recalls: "[T]here emerged from the woods a heavy line of the enemy's infantry and a battery on each flank, which opened fire on our advancing column and caused the brigade on our right to break, leaving our right flank entirely without protection. This compelled us to fall back across a field to a thicket of woods, where we rallied and in a few moments, with logs and fences, threw up a breastwork from which they did not try to dislodge us… "]*

May 9, 1864 - I am well at presant time. it is very hot.

May 10 - I am well at presant time. I am going to town to knight.

May 11 - I am well at presant time. it is a nice day.

May 12, 1864 - I am well at presant time. it is raining to day. *[On May 12, at the Bloody Angle near Spotsylvania, the 142ⁿᵈ Pennsylvania helps capture most of a division of Lee's army and nearly slices the Confederate army in two. Writes Warren: "The woods here were afire, and many of our wounded were burned to death, and when all was over and we landed behind our works once more, there were more than one of us expressed our thanks that we were alive and out of that place, which reminded us more of the infernal regions than any place we had yet had occasion to visit."]*

May 13 - I am well at presant time. it is raining to day. *[At the battle of Resaca, Georgia, Ephraim's cousin Daniel L. Minor of the 10ᵗʰ Ohio Cavalry is shot in the left thigh.]*

May 14 - I am well at presant time. it is a nice day. I am going to town to knight.

May 15, 1864 - I am well at presant time. it is raining to day.

May 16 - I am well at presant time. it is very warm.

May 17 - I am well at presant time.

May 18, 1864 - I am well at presant time. it is very warm.

May 19 - I am well at presant time. it is very warm and dry.

May 20 - I am well at presant time. it is very warm.

May 21, 1864 - I am well at presant time. it is very warm. I am going to the city.

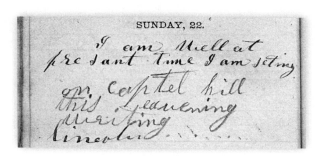

May 22 - I am well at presant time. I am seting on captel hill [Capitol Hill] this eavening writing. [Walt Whitman also is known to visit the capitol building occasionally, saying: "I like to stand aside and look a long, long while, up at the dome; it comforts me somehow."]

May 23 - I am well at presant time. [At North Anna River, the 142nd Pennsylvania continues to push toward Richmond. The move is stopped by Lee. Total casualties are 4,000. Writes Warren: "We had closed up our ranks and were marching in fours, expecting every moment the head of the column would halt, when, to the utter astonishment of all present, the enemy in a good solid line of battle emerged from the woods but a short distance from us, and commenced pouring into our ranks the

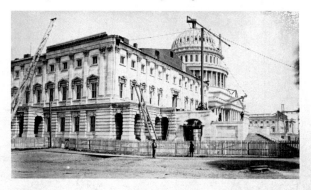

Unfinished U.S. Capitol dome in Washington, D.C., where Ephraim sat writing in his diary the evening of May 22, 1864. [Library of Congress]

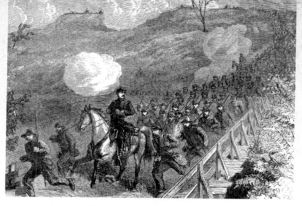

Union troops under fire at North Anna River, where the 142nd Pennsylvania was involved in action. [*Harper's Weekly*, June 25, 1864]

most murderous infantry fire I ever witnessed… A sheet of flame from our batteries and muskets not only checked the advancing enemy from driving us in the river, but sent them back over that field with as great, or greater, loss than we ourselves had sustained..."]

May 24, 1864 - I am well at presant time. it is a nice day.

May 25 - I am well at presant time. it is a very nice day. [*The 142nd Pennsylvania is at Jericho Ford.*]

May 26 - I am well at presant time. it is a nice day. [*The 142nd Pennsylvania is engaged in battle at Totopotomoy Creek. Warren writes: "[B]y reason of the stubbornness of the enemy's rear-guard, who sent us their compliments in the shape of shell and solid shot from their rearmost battery, we were forced into line of battle at Totopotomoy Creek, and our brigade pushed forward in line of battle for nearly a mile through the fields and woods. The result of which was the capture of about 100 tired-out Confederates, a cow and calf, some pigs, chickens and a barn full of tobacco."*]

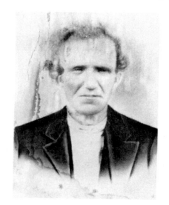

Chance Minor, Ephraim's younger brother, of the 1st West Virginia Cavalry.

May 27, 1864 - I am well at presant time. my brother came to see me to day. he is well. [*Ephraim likely is referring to his brother Chance Minor, who at the time is detached from the 1st West Virginia Cavalry and stationed in Alexandria, as a mounted orderly at*

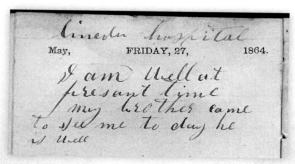

*the headquarters of Military Governor John P. Slough. In
addition to protecting the nation's capitol, Slough's charge is to
prevent the spread of smallpox and organize a camp to control
"convalescents, stragglers, and recruits."]*

May 28 - I am well at presant time. it is a nice day. *[The 142nd
Pennsylvania is in action at Totopotomoy Creek, facing an enemy
which has dug entrenchments along the creek. The inconclusive
fight forces the Union to withdraw back to Shady Grove Road.
Casualties suffered by both sides: 2,200.]*

May 29 - I am well at presant time. I am on capital hill at
present.

May 30, 1864 - I am well at presant time. I am white washing.

May 31, 1864 - I am well at presant time. I am white washing.

~ *June 1864* ~

June 1, 1864 - I am well at presant time I am white washing.
*[The 142nd Pennsylvania fights at "Second Cold Harbor" in
Virginia, including Bethesda Church. Some 170,000 forces
are involved, with 15,500 combined casualties, as Grant tries
to push ever-nearer to the heavily defended Richmond. In
Never Call Retreat, Catton says: "By now the armies were
running out of space. They had covered more than fifty miles
in the unmanageable, rolling series of battles that began in the
Wilderness, and now they could roll no more." After Union*

Fighting at Cold
Harbor, where the
142nd Pennsylvania
saw action. [*Harper's
Weekly*, June 25, 1864]

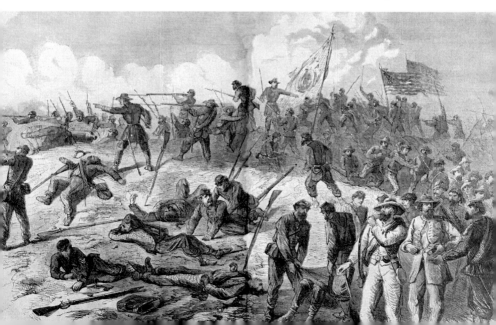

cavalry captures a key crossroads, the ensuing battle stretches along a seven-mile line. One Union assault is repulsed with heavy losses. Grant then makes the fateful decision to maneuver away from a direct assault on Richmond to focus instead on Petersburg.

Warren, of the 142nd Pennsylvania, recounts:
> *... early the next morning we found ourselves facing the same old enemy at Cold Harbor. Here they seemed to be in a terrible frame of mind and fought like wild cats. The losses in some of the new regiments to this battle, who were not accustomed to the bushwhacking warfare we had been engaged in for about three weeks, was simply terrible. The new regiments of heavy artillery that joined our army here, and were, by necessity, armed and used as infantry, were simply mowed down by the hundred, and fell and were swept to the earth almost like you have seen grain fall before the reaper. We hear that our watchword, "On to Richmond," was nearly realized, that we rejoiced in the belief that the city and Lee's whole force must soon succumb to the continued bull-dog persistence of our commander, General Grant, who, by this time, had given us to understand, and fully believe, that there would be no let up or cessation of hostilities until the desired end had been accomplished."]*

June 2, 1864 - I am well at presant time. I am white washing. *[At Cold Harbor, the 142nd Pennsylvania and Union forces are routed in the second day of battle. In Never Call Retreat, Catton says: "... a storm of Confederate rifle fire tore the Federal columns and inflicted a resounding defeat—the most unrelieved and tragically costly one the Army of the Potomac had suffered since it crossed the Rapidan..."]*

June 3 - I am well at presant time. I am slacking lime. *["Slacking lime" is a process of mixing water with lime to produce whitewash or a cement-like mortar.]*

June 4 - I am well at presant time. I am slacking lime.

June 5, 1864 - I am well at presant time. I am slacking lime.

June 6 - I am well at presant time. I am slacking lime.

June 7 - I am well at presant time. I am slacking lime.

June 8, 1864 - I am well at presant time. I am slacking lime.

[At the national convention of Republicans in Baltimore, President Lincoln is nominated for a second term.]

June 9 - I am well at presant time. I am slacking lime.

June 10 - I am well at presant time. I am slacking lime.

June 11, 1864 - I am well at presant time. I am slacking lime.

June 12 - I am well at presant time. it is very hout to day.

June 13 - I am well at presant time. I am working at my old traid *[trade]*.

June 14, 1864 - I am well at persant time. it is very hot.

June 15 - I am well at presant time. *[Robert E. Lee's former home and estate in Arlington, Virginia, now in the possession of the federals and in use as a burial ground, is signed into law as a national cemetery.]*

June 16 - I am well at presant time. it is very hout. *[The 142nd Pennsylvania is stationed at Petersburg. Having crossed the James River, the Union tries to press an assault on Petersburg, but is rebuffed with 4,500 losses. The army begins a siege around Petersburg that lasts for 10 months, from June 1864 to April 1865, with the 142nd Pennsylvania under fire every day for three months.]*

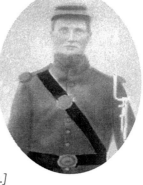

Robert Rankin, Ephraim's cousin by marriage, who was wounded at Petersburg.

June 17, 1864 - I am well at presant time. it is very hout.

June 18 - I am well at presant time. I am going to town to knight. *[During the Petersburg siege, Ephraim's cousin by marriage, Robert Rankin (husband of Hester Minerd), is shot in the leg during a charge.]*

June 19 - I am well at presant time. I am seeting *[sitting]* out on the capital hill writing this. I am going to meeting this after noon.

June 20, 1864 - I am well at present.

June 21 - I am well at present.

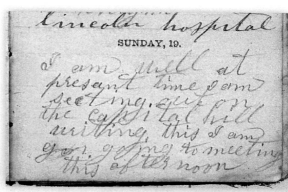

June 22 - I am well at present.

June 23, 1864 - I am well at presant time.

Friday 24 - I am well at presant time.

June 25 - I am well at present time. I am going out in the countery.

June 26, 1864 - I am well at presant time. I was out in the countery to day. I went down the directing [*direction of*] baltimore.

June 27 - I am well at presant time. it is very hot.

June 28 - I am well at presant time.

June 29, 1864 - I am well at presant time.

June 30 - I am well at present.

~ *July 1864* ~

July 1, 1864 - I am well at present. [*This is Ephraim's 26th birthday, but he does not mention it.*]

July 2, 1864 - I am well at presant time. it is a very nice day. [*Ephraim's cousin, Leroy Bush, dies at the home of his sister in Greenfield, Indiana, after contracting malaria as a member of the 9th Indiana Cavalry.*]

July 3 - I am well at presant time. I got a leter from Caroline. [*"Caroline" may be Caroline Schrock, a cousin on his mother's Younkin side of the family. In 1864, Ephraim receives seven letters from Caroline Schrock, as marked in the back of his diary.*]

July 4 - I am well at presant time. to day is forth of July. we have graite time in Washington.

July 5, 1864 - I am well at presant time. I am white washing to day.

July 6 - I am well at presant time. I am white washing to day. [*As a member of the 1st Maryland Cavalry, also known as the 1st Potomac Home Brigade Cavalry, Ephraim's future cousin by marriage, Richard Mason Gorsuch (husband of Martha Emma "Matt" Minerd), is shot on the left side of his stomach during a nighttime charge at Maryland Heights, near Harper's Ferry.*]

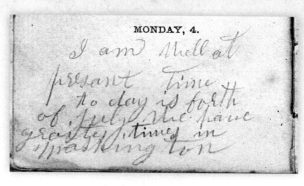

MONDAY, 4.

I am well at presant time to day is forth of July the have grateyst times in washington

July 7 - I am well at presant time. I am white washing.

July 8, 1864 - I am well at presant time. I am white washing.

July 9 - I am not well. I am doing nothing. [*At the battle of Monocacy Junction, Maryland, Ephraim's cousin Eli Van Horn, of the 144th Ohio Infantry, is shot through his breast, but survives.*]

July 10 - I am no beter. I have a bad cole.

Fourth of July celebrations in Civil War camps. [*Harper's Weekly*, July 1861]

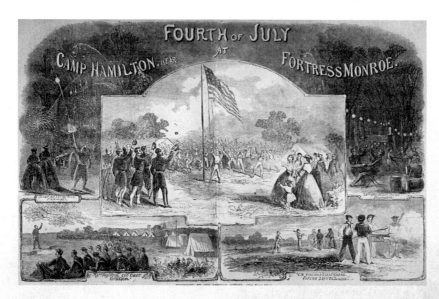

FOURTH OF JULY

CAMP HAMILTON, NEAR AT FORTRESS MONROE.

Camp near fort slocum

Camp - near fort slocum

I am well at present
time this mourning
I left the hospital and
Went to fort slocum

Camp near fort Slocum

TUESDAY, 12.

I am well at presa[...]
the fight has begun
fort stephant and
fort slocum
opent on the rebels
and fort Lounker
ane fort Lahill

WEDNESDAY, 13.

I am well at
present We are
at fort stephants
the rebels left

July 11, 1864 - I am
well at present time.
this mourning I left the
hospital and went to
fort slocum. *[Stevens
and Slocum are among a
ring of forts protecting our
nation's capital during the
war. Stevens (also spelled
"Stephens"), sits along a
strategic approach to the
city near today's Walter
Reed Army Hospital.
Also on July 10, Grant
creates a large supply
center and hospital at the
confluence of the James and
Appomattox Rivers, known
as City Point, a waterway
deep within Virginia that
contains important railway
connections to key southern
cities. Ephraim would
spend time at City Point
in December 1864 and in*

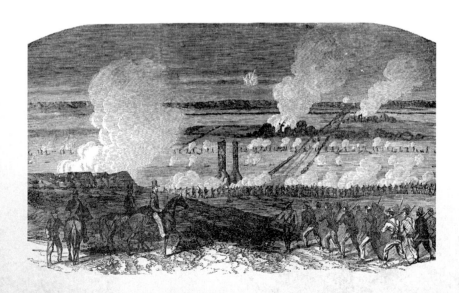

Janaury, February and April 1865.]

July 12 - I am well at present. the fight has begun. fort stephant and fort slocum opent on the rebels and fort bounker and fort la hill. *[The battle at Fort Stevens is the only one to take place within the District of Columbia, and the first to be viewed firsthand by President Lincoln. In* Abraham Lincoln: The War Years, *Carl Sandburg describes this battle: "For the first time in his life Abraham Lincoln saw men in battle action go to their knees and sprawl on the earth with cold lead in their vitals, with holes plowed by metal through their heads... Now for the first time he saw them as the rain of enemy rifle shots picked them off." In this unprotected moment, an enemy bullet "whizzes" no more than five feet from Lincoln's head. Yelps a nearby officer, "Get down, you fool!"]*

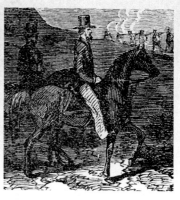

Opposite page: Fighting at Fort Stevens, near Washington, D.C., which Ephraim witnessed, as did President Lincoln (above, on a horse, wearing a highly visible top hat). *[Scenes And Portraits Of The Civil War]*

July 13 - I am well at present. we are at fort stephants. the rebels left.

July 14, 1864 - I am well at presant time. we are at fort stephants yet. *[Ephraim's cousin by marriage, William J. Burditt (husband of Jemima Minerd), is released from a Confederate prison after 13 months as a POW.]*

July 15 - I am well at presant time. we are at the fort yet.

July 16 - I am well at present time. we are stil at fort slocum.

July 17, 1864 - I am well at presant time. it is very warm.

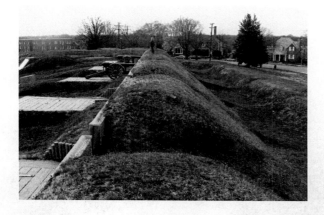

Site of Fort Stevens today, Rock Creek Park on Georgia Avenue and Quackenbos Street in the District of Columbia, near Walter Reed Army Medical Center. [Author photo.]

Camp clifton barrock [Barracks]

July 18 - I am well at presant this after noon we left camp and went to clifton barack. *[Clifton Barracks is across the street from the White House, to the south. While Ephraim never mentions seeing the president, Walt Whitman writes of glimpsing Lincoln "almost every day."]*

July 19 - I am well at presant time.

July 20, 1864 - I am well at presant time. it is very hot today.

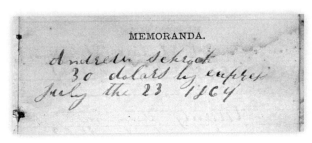

July 21 - I am well at presant time. I sind *[signed]* the pay roles to day.

July 22 - I am well at presant time.

July 23, 1864 - I am well at presant time I got paid off yesterday.

Payday for Union soldiers. [*The Civil War in the United States*]

[In the back of the diary is this inscription about money Ephraim sends home to the care of his uncle: "Memoranda—Andrew Schrock 30 dolars by express July the 23 1864."]

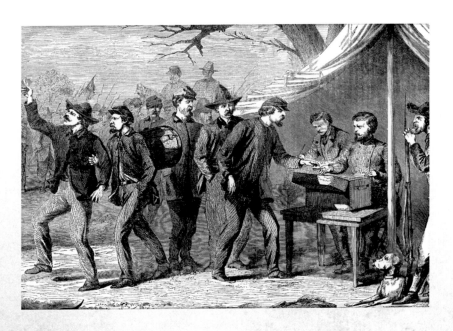

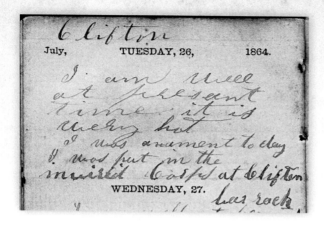

July 24 - I am well at present. I am going to leave lincoln hospital this morning and go to Cliften barrack.

July 25 - I am well at presant time. I am at Clifton. I think I am going to the regiment in a few days.

July 26, 1864 - I am well at presant time. it is very hot. I was axament *[examined]* to day. I was put in the invalid corps at Cliften barrack. *[See the entry of Oct. 17, 1864, when Ephraim officially is assigned to the Invalid Corps, and joins the 22nd Regiment, Veteran Reserve Corps (VRC). This signifies the Army's belief that he remains unfit for active duty, but with prolonged recovery might at least furnish valuable light duty service, freeing up more able-bodied men for more important tasks elsewhere. The VRC is created during the war to employ "worthy" convalescing and disabled soldiers in tasks such as guard duty and hospital aides. Some 60,000 disabled Union soldiers eventually serve with the corps during the war.]*

July 27 - I am well at presant time. it is very hot.

July 28 - I am well at presant time.

July 29, 1864 - I am well at presant time. it is very hot.

July 30 - I am well at presant time. it is very hot and dry. *[The 142nd Pennsylvania is on duty near Petersburg when an ill-planned Union mine detonates in tunnels underneath the Confederate lines. At this battle, Ephraim's cousin by marriage, John Strauch (husband of Mary Hester McKnight) is deafened by "heavy cannonading" with the 155th Pennsylvania Infantry. This blunder later is featured in the film, Cold Mountain.]*

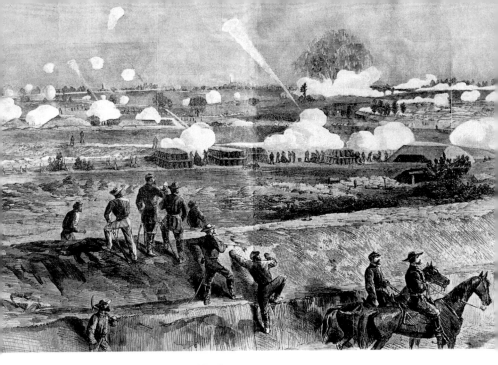

Petersburg—massive explosion of the underground mine and disastrous assault. [*Harper's Weekly*, Aug. 20, 1864]

Of this debacle, Warren writes:

> *The lines all along for about five miles were in readiness at 4 a.m., and when the torch was lighted which blew up the mine, all the artillery, numbering several hundred guns, and all the infantry with their muskets let loose at one time. It made a lively commotion among our enemies, who, with the exception of their picket, were quietly sleeping. Had a charge been made right away after this bombardment and tremendous volley, I have no doubt Petersburgh and the entire Army of Northern Virginia under Lee would have been captured, for the ground shook for miles around almost as if an earthquake had taken place, and prisoners which we took afterwards informed us that on that morning for a few moments their entire line was paralyzed with fear lest they should all be hurled in the air and buried in a similar way to those in the fort that was blown up.]*

July 31 - I am well at presant time. I was put in the invirlid core [*Invalid Corps*] this after noon.

~ August 1864 ~

Aug. 1, 1864 - I am well at presant time. I left Cliften barracks this eavening and went to the avenue near george town on 22 street. *[Ephraim is assigned to Cliffburne Hospital in the Meridian Hill section of District of Columbia. Cliffburne once housed Confederate prisoners, but now treats Union troops. With 15,000 Confederate troops under Jubal Early threatening the outskirts of Washington, Ephraim and VRC troops are ordered to the city's defenses. Also in August, Ephraim's brother Chance, an orderly in Alexandria, is treated for chronically loose bowels.]*

Camp fry Washington
[Camp Fry is a post hospital for VRC troops.]

Aug. 2 - I am well at present time. it is very hot and dry. *[Ephraim's cousin, Andrew Jackson Miner of the 90th Ohio Volunteer Infantry (not to be confused with Ephraim's brother of the same name), dies of severe diarrhea at Vining Station, Georgia, during Sherman's Atlanta campaign.]*

Aug. 3 - I am well at presant time. I was on inspecting to day. I got a nu *[new]* gun to day.

Aug. 4, 1864 - I am well at presant time. I am going on a pass today. I am going to the lincoln hospital to see som of the old boys.

Aug. 5 - I am well at presant time. I was out drilling this mourning.

Aug. 6 - I am well at presant time. I am doing nothing do day.

Aug. 7, 1864 - I am well at presant time. we had a inspecting this mourning and very clost *[close?]*.

Aug. 8 - I am well at presant time. I was out on drill this mourning. it is very hot and dry.

Aug. 9 - I am well at presant time. I was out on drill this mourning. it is very hot and dry.

Aug. 10, 1864 - I am well at presant time. I was out on drill this mourning. it is very hot. I am going out on a pass this eavening. I am a going to have som foune *[some fun]*.

Aug. 11 - I am well at presant time. I was out on drill this mourning. it is ofle *[awful]* hot. we nearly rost *[roast]* up but we have good time.

Aug. 12 - I am well at presant time I am doing nothing to day it is very hot.

Aug. 13, 1964 - I am well at presant time. I am on gard today on 18 street. it is ofel hot but we had a good raine this after noon. it is cule and nice. *[While guarding a rail line in Berryville, Virginia, Ephraim's cousin Isaac Van Horn, of the 144th Ohio Infantry, is captured and later taken to POW camps in Richmond.]*

Aug. 14 - I am well at presant time. I got of gard *[off guard]* this mourning. it is very hot and I am very lasey to day.

[Ephraim's cousin, James Minerd Jr., of the 85th Pennsylvania Infantry, is shot in the leg at Deep Bottom/ Strawberry Plains, Virginia.]

August,   TUESDAY, 16,   1864.

Aug. 15 - I am well at presant time. I am doing nothing to day. it is very hout but we had a good raine this after noon.

Aug. 16, 1864 - I am not well. I have the rhumetism in my legs and feet. I am on gard today. it gows very hard to stan gard. it raind very hard this after noon.

Aug. 17 - I am beter to day. we had a inspecting of armes this after noon. this after noon it raind very hard this after noon.

Aug. 18 - I am well at presant time. I was out on drill this mouring *[morning]*. it is raining this mourning. it is very warm. I am going to town this after noon. *[Continuing in the months' long siege around Petersburg, the 142nd Pennsylvania takes part in action at the Weldon Railroad. This is part of Grant's continuing maneuvers at Petersburg to put pressure on Richmond, and Union forces succeed in cutting off the railroad line.]*

Aug. 19, 1864 - I am well at presant time. I am doing nothing to day. it is raining it is very whet this to weakes *[two weeks]*.

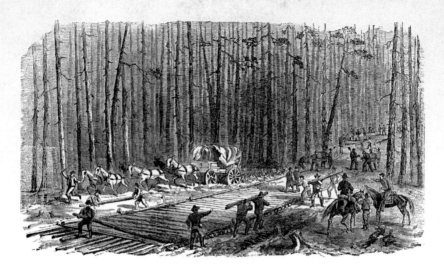

Aug. 20 - I am well at presant time. I am on gard at george town. it is raining to day. [*At Jonesboro, Georgia, Ephraim's cousin Frederick Miner Jr. is injured when his horse is shot and the soldier is thrown from the saddle, suffering a severe hernia.*]

Construction of a plank road during the assault on the prized Weldon Railroad [*The Civil War in the United States*]

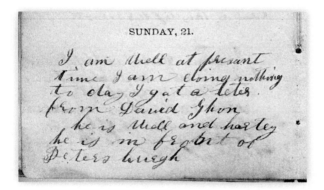

Aug. 21 - I am well at presant time. I am doing nothing to day. I got a leter from David Ghon. he is well and hartey [*hearty*]. he is in front of Peteres burgh. [*Ghon, a.k.a. "Gohn," is a corporal in the 142nd Pennsylvania. He later is wounded at Hatchers' Run/Dabney's Mills. See entry for Feb. 5, 1865.*]

Aug. 22, 1864 - I am well at presant time. I am on gard to day. it is raining this mourning. I am on gard on 18 street.

Aug. 23 - I am well at presant time. I am doing nothing to day. it is very hot. I am going out on a pass this eavening on a short. I am very lasey this after noon.

Aug. 24 - I am well at presant time. I am doing nothing to day. it is very warm and I am very lasey.

Aug. 25, 1864 - I am well at present time. I am on gard to day. it is raining to day.

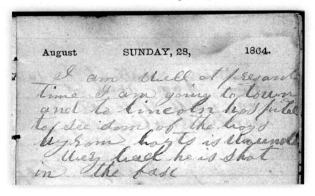

Aug. 26 - I am well at presant time. I am doing nothing to day. it is very hot to day. I am very lasey.

Aug. 27 - I am well at presant time. I am on gard at george town. it is very hot to day.

Aug. 28, 1864 - I am well at presant time. I am going to town and to lincoln hospital to see som of the boys. hyram boyts is wounded very bad. he is shot in the fase. [*Hiram Boyts, a private in the 142nd Pennsylvania, is mortally wounded at Petersburg. He dies in Washington, D.C. on the very day Ephraim writes this entry. Several of Boyts' war letters are on file at the Historical and Genealogical Society of Somerset County, Pennsylvania.*]

Aug. 29 - I am well at presant time. I am on gard to day at george town.

Aug. 30 - I am well at presant time. I am doing nothing to day.

Aug. 31, 1864 - I am well at presant time. I was musterd to day. I think we will go a way this after noon or tomorrow. we will go to new york or to philadelphia. [*At the national convention of Democrats in Chicago, former Union General McClellan is nominated for the presidency.*]

~ September 1864 ~

Sept. 1, 1864 - I am well at presant time. I am on gard to day on the aven new [*avenue*] on 18 street and on 19 street. we have marching orders. it is very cule [*cool*] at knight.

Sept. 2 - I am well at presant time. I am on gard to day at george town. it is very hot.

Sept. 3 1864 - I am well at presant time. I am doing nothing to day. I am going out on a pass this after noon.

Sept. 4 - I am very well at presant time. I am on gard to day at george town. we left and went to camp for to go to new york. We are a going to leave.

Sept. 5 - I am well at present time. I am doing nothing to day. I am very lasey [lazy]. it is very warm. we are going to leave this eavening at 9 oclock.

Sept. 6, 1864 - I am well at presant time. we are in philadelphia at present. I just had my super [supper]. we are a going on the boat in a few minets to go to new york.

> September, TUESDAY, 6, 1864.
>
> I am well at presant time the are in philadelphia at presant. I just had my super the are a going on the boat in a few minets to go to new york
>
> WEDNESDAY, 7.
>
> I am well at presant time the are noll in Jersey jersey city

Union soldiers boarding the train in the Jersey City depot. [Scenes And Portraits Of The Civil War]

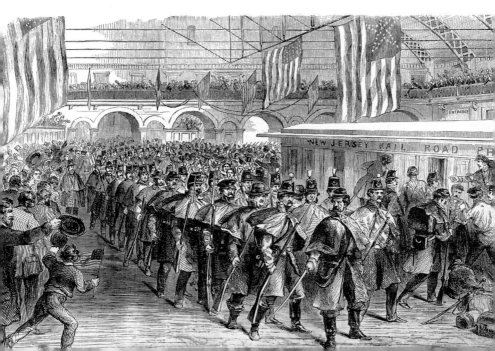

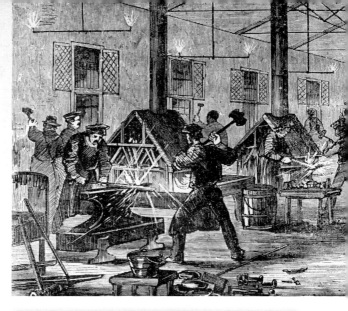

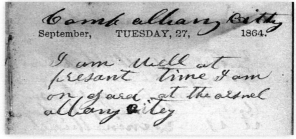

September,   TUESDAY, 27,   1864.

Camp albany citty

I am well at presant time I am on guard at the arsnel albany citty

Shipment of guns and ammunition from the arsenal near Albany. [*The Civil War in the United States*]

Sept. 7 - I am well at presant time. we are now in new jursey city.

Camp albany citty [*Ephraim and the 22nd VRC are assigned to guard a large federal arsenal along the Hudson River six miles north of Albany. The arsenal employs 1,500 men, and a history*

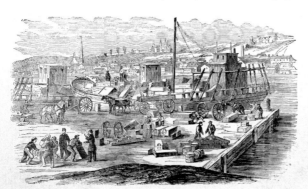

of the region says that work "continued day and night to fill the requisitions for ordnance supplies for our armies during their continuous engagements." The 22nd VRC remains in Albany for a little more than three weeks.]

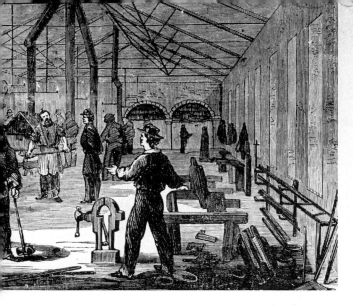

Federal arsenal at Watevliet near Albany, New York, forging ironwork for gun carriages, which Ephraim helped guard in late September 1864. [*The Civil War in the United States*]

Sept. 8 - I am well at presant time we are know [*now*] in the stat of new york, houlliney [*?*] city. I think we will stay hear this winter.

Sept. 9, 1864 - I am well at presant time. I am doing nothing to day. I lik this plase very well. I am going to town to albany city.

Sept. 10 - I am well at presant time. I am doing nothing do day.

Sept. 11 - I am well at presant time. I am on gard to day. it is very cold.

Sept. 12, 1864 - I am well at presant. I am doing nothing today. I was in town to day. it is very cold and cloudy.

Sept. 13 - I am well at presant time. I am going to town to day. it is very cold.

Sept. 14 - I am well, only my leg paines very much. it is cule. I am doing nothing to day.

Sept. 15, 1864 - I am well at presant. I am doing nothing to day. is it very nice day.

> Camp Albany N.
> WEDNESDAY, 14.
> I am well only
> my leg paines very
> much it is cule
> I am doing nothing
> to day

Sept. 16 - I am well at presant time. I am doing nothing to day. it is a very nice day.

Sept. 17 - I am well at presant time. I am on gard to day at albany city. it is cold and it is raining this mourning.

Sept. 18, 1864 - I am well at present time. I am doing nothing to day. I am very lone som today. I had a dreem last knight that I was at home discharge. it was a small *[illegible]* to me.

Sept. 19 - I am well at presant time. I am doing nothing to day. it is a very nice day. very warm.

Sept. 20 - I am well at presant time. I am doing nothing.

Sept. 21, 1864 - I am doing nothing to day. I am well at presant time. only drill a litle som times.

Sept. 22 - I am well at presant time. I am on gard to day. it is very cule.

Sept. 23 - I am well at presant time. I am doing nothing to day. it is very windey.

Sept. 24, 1864 - I am well at presant time. I am doing nothing to day. it is very winday to day. it is raining this after noon. *[At Kennesaw Mountain (Big Shanty), Georgia, Ephraim's cousin Samuel Miner, of the 19th Ohio Infantry, is captured and later held at Andersonville Prison.]*

Sept. 25 - I am well at presant time. I am doing nothing to day. it is very cold.

Sept. 26 - I am well at this time. I am doing nothing today. it is a very nice day.

Sept. 27, 1864 - I am well at presant time. I am on gard at the arsnel albany city.

Sept. 28 - I am well at presant time. I just got off gard. I am doing nothing this afternoon. it is a very nice day.

Sept. 29 - I am well at presant time. I am doing nothing to day. I am going to the city this eavening. *[The 142nd Pennsylvania is at Poplar Springs Church and Peeble's Farm near the Weldon Railroad, south of Petersburg. Seeking to keep pressing toward Richmond, Grant launches his fifth offensive of the siege. With Lee primarily engaged north of Petersburg,*

Grant's army successfully captures important supply routes and communications lines to the south and west of the city.]

Sept. 30, 1864 - I am well at presant time. I am doing nothing to day.

~ October 1864 ~

Oct. 1, 1864 - I am well at presant time. I am doing nothing to day. I was payd off this after noon. We are a going to leave this camp.

Oct. 2 - I am well at presant time. I am doing nothing this mourning. we left albany and start to india *[Indiana].*

Oct. 3, 1864 - I am well at presant time. we are in buflow *[Buffalo, New York].* it is 10 oclock. we are a going leave at 11 oclock.

Oct. 4 - I am well at presant time. we are in india state indinpls *[Indiana state, Indianapolis. Ephraim and the 22nd VRC are sent here to guard a prisoner of war camp and provide guard and orderly services at a local hospital and soldiers' home. They remain in Indiana until December 10.]*

Oct. 5 - I am well at presant time. we are a going to leave this plase this eavening and go to Mishigan citty Indianania *[Michigan City, Indiana].*

The Union railroad depot in Indianapolis, where Ephraim arrived in the city. [Engraved by Howe Barber, 1861]

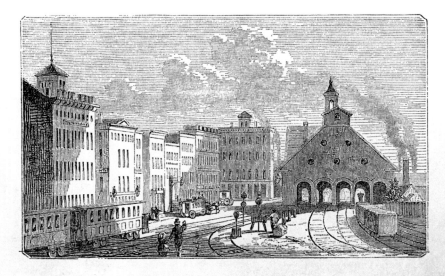

Oct. 6, 1864 - I am well at presant time. we are stil going north.

Oct. 7 - I am well at presant time. we are stil going north.

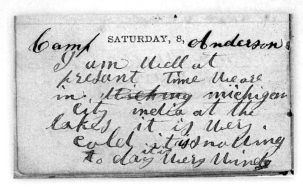

Camp Anderson, Michigan

Oct. 8 - I am well at presant time. we are in michigan city inda at the lakes. it is very cold. it is snowing to day. very windy. [*Camp Anderson earlier is a training ground for Indiana regiments and later houses VRC trooops.*]

Oct. 9, 1864 - I am well at present time. it is very cold to day.

Oct. 10 - I am well at present. I am doing nothing to day. it is very cold.

Oct. 11 - I am well at presant time.

Oct. 12, 1864 - I am well at presant time. I am on duty. I am ordley [*orderly*].

Wartime military hospital in Indianapolis, where Ephraim likely served as an orderly.

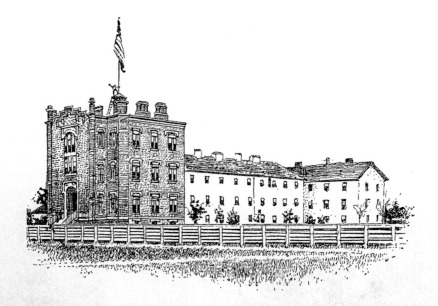

Oct. 13 - I am well at presant time. I am doing nothing to day.

Oct. 14 - I am well at presant time. it is very cold.

Oct. 15, 1864 - I am well at presant time. it is cold. I am on gard to day.

Oct. 16 - I am well at presant time. it is cold. I am doing nothing to day.

Oct. 17 - I am well at presant time. I am on gard to day. it is cold to day. *[Having continuously accrued pay from the 142nd Pennsylvania during his convalescence, but still not fit for duty, Ephraim officially is transferred to the 22nd Veterans Reserve Corps. Many thousands of men join the VRC and are moved to vital locations throughout the northern states, providing light duty services as guards at POW camps and arsenals and as hospital orderlies. Also see entry of July 26, 1864.]*

Oct. 18, 1864 - I am well at presant time. I am doing nothing today.

Oct. 19 - I am well at presant time. I am on gard to day. it is cold.

Oct. 20 - I am well at presant time. I am doing nothing to day. it is a very nice day.

Oct. 21, 1864 - I am well at presant time. I am on gard to day.

Oct. 22 - I am well at presant time. I am doing nothing to day. it is a nice day. I am going to town.

Oct. 23 - I am well at presant time. I am doing nothing to day. it is a very nice day.

Oct. 24, 1864 - I am well at presant time. I am on gard to day. it is a nice day.

Oct. 25 - I am well at presant time. I am doing nothing to day. it is very cold.

Oct. 26 - I am well at presant time. I am going to Indianania Citty *[Indianapolis]* with some subes *[subs – "substitutes"]*

Oct. 27, 1864 - I am well at presant time. I am in the citty of Indianiania. we are going to go back to mishig citty *[Michigan City]* this eavening. *[The 142nd Pennsylvania is at Boydton Plank Road and Hatcher's Run, Virginia. There, 35,000 troops under Union Major General Winfield Scott Hancock and Confederate Major General Henry Heth face each other, with 3,058 combined casualties. Continuing to maneuver around the stalemated Petersburg, Hancock's forces capture the Boydton Plank Road, but they abandon it again after an enemy counterattack.]*

Oct. 28 - I am well at presant time. I got back to old camp this mourning about 6 oclock.

Oct. 29 - I am well at presant time. I am doing nothing today. it is raining to day.

Oct. 30, 1864 - I am well at present time. I am on gard today. it is a nice day.

Oct. 31 - I am well at presant time. I am going to town. it is very nice day.

~ November 1864 ~

Nov. 1 - I am well at presant time. I am doing nothing to day. *[In November, Ephraim's brother Chance is again treated in a hospital in Alexandria for severely loose bowels.]*

Nov. 2, 1864 - I am well at presant time. I am on gard to day. it is could *[cold]*.

Nov. 3 - I am well at presant time. I am going to town.

Nov. 4 - I am well at presant time. it is snowing do day. it is very cold.

Nov. 5, 1864 - I am not very well. I am ofle *[awful]* sore. I cant harley *[hardly]* walk. the snow is all gone a way.

Nov. 6 - I am well at presant time. I am doing nothing to day. it is raining to day. I am going to town this after noon.

Nov. 7 - I am not well to day. I am very sick. it is a nice day.

Nov. 8, 1864 - I am well at presant time. it is raining to day. it is lecking *[election]* day today. *[Lincoln is re-elected for a second term as President of the United States, with 55 percent of the popular vote.]*

Nov. 9 - I am very sick but I am giting beter. it is very cold.

Nov. 10 - I am beter this mourning. it is very cold.

Nov. 11, 1864 - I am stil giting beter. it is very cold. pritey good snow on the ground.

Camp Anderson Michigan Citty Indianania

Nov. 12 - I am beter this mourning. it is very cold. the snow is a half foot deep. it is stil snowing.

Nov. 13 - I am a bout well a gaine. it haint very cold to day but the snow is a bout a foot deep.

Nov. 14, 1864 - I am well at presant time. I am on gard to day. it is raining to day.

Nov. 15 - I am well at presant time. I am going to the citty. it is nice day. [*Having captured Atlanta, General William Tecumseh Sherman launches a four-month march through Georgia which results in widespread destruction throughout the state.*]

Ephraim's cousin and correspondent Joanna (Minerd) Enos and her husband Perry.

Nov. 16 - I am well at presant time. I am doing nothing to day. it is raining to day.

Nov. 17, 1864 - I am well at presant time. I am doing nothing to day. it is raining to day. I got a leter from joanna this mourning. I was very glad. [*The writer "Joanna" likely is either his future wife Joanna Younkin or his first cousin Joanna Minerd, from whom he is received 17 letters during the year, as marked in the back of the 1864 diary. After the war, Joanna Minerd marries Perry Enos, a veteran of the 188th Pennsylvania Infantry.*]

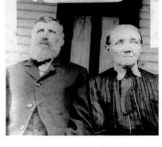

Nov. 18 - I am well at presant time. I am doing nothing to day. it is a very nice day to day.

Nov. 19 - I am well at presant time. I am going to the citty.

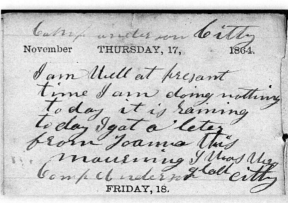

Camp Anderson Citty
November THURSDAY, 17, 1864.

I am Well at presant time I am doing nothing to day it is raining to day I got a leter from Joanna this mauring I was Ue Camp Anderson glad citty

FRIDAY, 18.

Nov. 20, 1864 - I am well at presant time. I am doing nothing to day. it is a very nice day.

Nov. 21 - I am well at presant time. I am doing nothing to day. it is very cold. the snow is about half foot deep.

Nov. 22 - I am well at presant time. I am on tig *[fatigue duty?]* today. it is very cold.

Nov. 23, 1864 - I am well at presant time. I am on gard to day. I got paid off this mourning. it is very cold.

Nov. 24 - I am well at presant time. I am going to the citty this day. it is very nice day.

Nov. 25 - I am well at presant time. I am doing nothing to day. it is raining to day. the snow is nearley all gone a way.

Nov. 26, 1864 - I am well at presant time. I am doing nothing to day. it is a nice day.

Nov. 27 - I am well at presant time. I am doing nothing to day. it is raining to day.

Nov. 28 - I am well at present time. I am going to town to day. it is raining.

Nov. 29, 1864 - I am well at presant time. I am doing nothing to day. it is a very nice day.

Nov. 30 - I am well at presant time. I am doing nothing to day. it is a very nice day.

~ December 1864 ~

Dec. 1 - I am well at presant time. I am doing nothing to day. it is a very nice day.

Dec. 2, 1864 - I am well at presant time. we are a going to leave this Camp at 10 oclock this mourning.

Dec. 3 - I am well at presant time. we are in the city of Indianopiles

SATURDAY, 3.

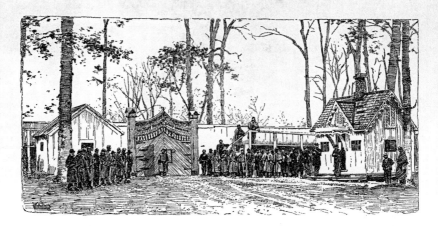

but we are a going to Camp bournes sides ["Camp Burnside" is near the Camp Morton POW camp on what is now 16th Street in Indianapolis. VRC troops guard thousands of POWs at Morton. Rumors abound—and later are disproved—that conditions are so poor that VRC guards freeze to death while on duty during wintry nights. Observing these camps, the U.S. Christian Commission says that the veterans "are the made of sterling stuff: their duties have been exceedingly arduous and responsible."]

Front gate at Camp Morton, near Indianapolis, which held POWs during the war, and where Ephraim likely served as a guard in October 1864. [The Century Magazine, 1891]

Dec. 4 - I am not very well at presant time. we are at souldiers home at presant time but we are a going a way this eavening or tomorrow mourning. [The soldiers home in Indianapolis, at the corner of West and Maryland streets, lodges tens of thousands of men. According to Indianapolis and the Civil War, "So many soldiers were continually passing through the city or remaining for a short time, both in bodies and individually, and for whom camps were not suitable, that it was absolutely necessary to provide a place for them."]

Dec. 5, 1864 - I am well at presant time. we are stil at souldiers home. we are expect [expected] to go a way every day. it is a nice day.

Dec. 6 - I am well at presant time. We are still at souldiers home. it is cloudy to day and could [cold].

Dec. 7 - I am well at presant time. we are stil at souldiers home and nothing to do. it raind last knight. it is could. [The 142nd Pennsylvania is part of another expedition to Weldon Railroad. Warren writes: "... their losses were very heavy, ours

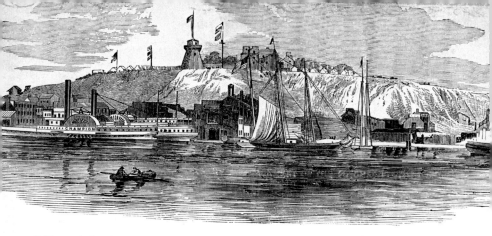

Baltimore during the war. [*The Civil War in the United States*]

slight. *Here we realized the difference between offensive and defensive warfare. Behind our works we felt secure, and when they came out and charged us three lines deep, we literally mowed them down."]*

Dec. 8, 1864 - I am well at presant time. we are stil at souldiers home. it is very cold. we nearly froze last night.

Dec. 9 - I am well at presant time. we are stil at souldiers home, yet it is very cold. we are under marching orders. we are going to baultimore citty [Baltimore, Maryland].

Dec. 10 - I am well at presant time. we are a going to leave this eavening for baultimore. we are on the traine. the snow is a [illegible].

Dec. 11, 1864 - I am well at presant time. we are in ohio at presant time. we are in pitts burgh at present. we go hear at 5 oclock. we had a good souper [supper].

Dec. 12 - I am well at presant time. we left pitts

burgh this mourning at three oclock. we are in altonah
[*Altoona, Pennsylvania*]. it is very cold. the snow is a bout half
foot deep.

Dec. 13 - I am well at presant time. we are in baultimore
citty. we pass threw jonns town yesterday. I wod like to
com home when I was at johnes town. [*Johnstown, Cambria
County, Pennsylvania is about 50 miles from Ephraim's home
at Kingwood.*]

Camp Bradford Baltimore

Dec. 14, 1864 - I am well at presant time. I am doing nothing
to day. it a nice day. [*Camp Bradford is a post hospital near
Baltimore, with the capacity to serve 1,000 invalids. It is located
on North Charles Street "on the grounds of the former State
Agricultural Society, where the State, Cattle and miscellaneous
Fairs were held for many years," says the U.S. Christian
Commission in a report. "The situation is high and healthy, and
possesses many attractions from the beauty of the position and its
proximity to some of the finest and most elegant residences and
farms in Baltimore county."*]

Dec. 15 - I am well at presant time. it is very could today. I am
doing nothing to day.

Dec. 16 - I am well at presant time. I am on gard to day. it
raining to day. [*Ephraim's future nephew by marriage, Cyrus
Lindley (husband of Elizabeth Miner), of the 140th Pennsylvania
Infantry, is released after being held in Southern prisons in
Richmond and Andersonville.*]

Dec. 17, 1864 - I am well at presant time. I am going to town
this after noon. it is cloudy and not very cold.

Dec. 18 - I am well at presant time. I am going to Washington
Citty this after noon. gard draftet men [*guard drafted men*].

Dec. 19 - I am well at presant time. I am going to city point
this after noon with substitute. it is very mudy. it is raining
to day.

Dec. 20, 1864 - I am well at presant time. we are on the
James river going to citty point. we are at fortes monrow
[*Fortress Monroe*]. we are a going to leave at 11 oclock.
[*Fortress Monroe is located at Hampton, Virginia. It serves
as the headquarters of the Union Army during the siege of*

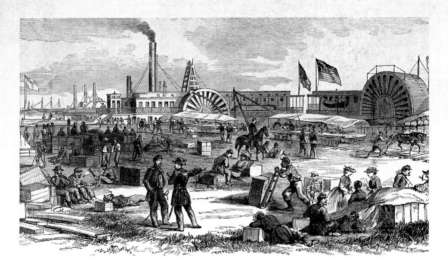

Reception of wounded Union soldiers at Fortress Monroe, with cars carrying them to the hospital. [From a sketch by Schell, 1890]

Petersburg. Two years earlier, Ephraim's cousin Leonard Rowan, of the the 85th Pennsylvania Infantry, dies at the fort's hospital after suffering from over exertion and fatigue. In 1865, former Confederate President Jefferson Davis is imprisoned at the fort, and held for two years.]

Dec. 21 - I am well at presant time. we are at citty point. we are a going to stay all night. it is very cold.

Dec. 22 - I am well at presant time. we are going to leave this eavening for the secent [Second] Corps. it is very cold and windy. it is very quite loung [quiet along] the lines this eavening. we are back to citty point.

Dec. 23, 1864 - I am well at presant time. we are a going to leave city point this mourning for baltimore.

Dec. 24 - I am well at presant time. we got to baltimore this mourning at 8 oclock. the snow is a bout one half foot deep. it is not very cold.

Dec. 25 - [Christmas Day] I am well at presant time. I am doing nothing to day. it is a nice day. the snow is one half foot deep. it is going a way.

Dec. 26, 1864 - I am well at this time. I am going to citty point this after noon.

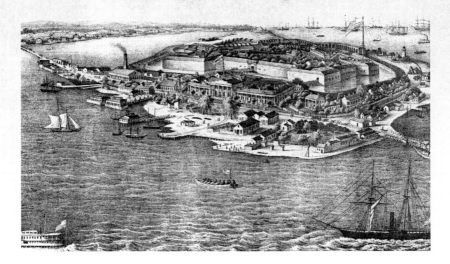

Dec. 27 - I am well at this time. we are at fortes monro at this time.

Dec. 28 - I am well at this time. we are at city point. we are a going to start for Baltimore.

Dec. 29, 1864 - I am well at this time. I am back to camp a gaine. we have very good times.

Dec. 30 - I am well at this time. it is very cold at this time.

Dec. 31 - I am well at this time. it is very cold at this time. this is the last day of this mounth.

Fortress Monroe, where Ephraim arrived five days before Christmas 1864, and where his cousin Leonard Rowan had died of "paralysis" 16 months earlier. [Lithograph by Edward Sachse & Co., Baltimore. Published by C. Bohn, Washington, D.C., 1862]

PART V

The Diary for 1865

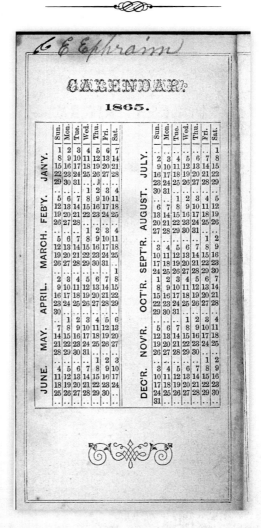

~ January 1865 ~

Jan. 1, 1865 - Camp Bradford Baltimore - I am well at this time. I am on guard today. it is very cold to day.

Jan. 2 - I am well at this time. it is very cold. the snow is about too inches deep.

Jan. 3 - I am well at this time. it is a nice day.

Jan. 4, 1865 - Camp Bradford Baltimore - I am well at this time. it is very cold. it is snowing too day.

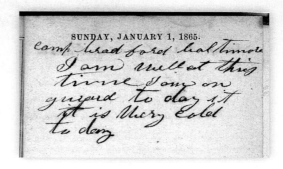

SUNDAY, JANUARY 1, 1865.

Jan. 5 - I am well at this time. it is very cold.

Jan. 6 - I am well at this time. it is very cold to day.

Jan. 7, 1865 - Camp Bradford Baltimore - I am well at this time. it is very cold.

Jan. 8 - I am well at this time. it is cold and it is raining.

Jan. 9 - I am well at this time. it is very cold to day. *[While accompanying substitute soldiers on a march, Ephraim and Frederick Braun of the 22nd VRC, and perhaps others, are confined in the hands of military authorities in Baltimore on charges of "defrauding" their escorts. The details are not known. Ephraim's official military record only contains a brief mention, and the diary is entirely silent on the matter. While in custody, and the charges investigated, Ephraim provides guard duty and travels to and from City Point and Fortress Monroe. On many of the days, however, he is idle. Ephraim and Braun are released and return to duty after a little more than two months, on March 18.]*

Jan. 10, 1865 - Camp Bradford Baltimore - I am well at this time. it is very cold to day.

Jan. 11 - I am well at this time. is cold and winday. *[Ephraim's cousin Alpheus Minerd, and Minerd's*

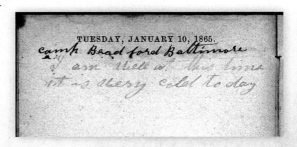

TUESDAY, JANUARY 10, 1865.

brother-in-law William H. Shepard, both of the 34th Ohio Infantry, are captured in action at Beverly, West Virginia.]

Jan. 12 - I am well at this time. it is very cold.

Jan. 13, 1865 - Camp Bradford Baltimore - I am well at this time. it is very cold to day.

Jan. 14 - I am well at this time. it is very cold to day.

Jan. 15 - I am well at this time. it is very cold.

Jan. 16, 1865 - Camp Bradford Baltimore - I am well at this time. it is very cold to day. I am going to city point.

Jan. 17 - I am well at this time. it is very cold to day.

Jan. 18 - I am well at this time. it is very cold to day.

Jan. 19, 1865 - Camp Bradford Baltimore - I am well at this time. it is a nice day.

Jan. 20 - I am well at this time. it is a nice day. I am doing nothing.

Jan. 21 - I am well at this time.

Jan. 22, 1865 - I am well at this time. it is a nice day.

Jan. 23 - I am well at this time. it is very cold.

Jan. 24 - I am well at this time.

Jan. 25, 1865 - I am well at this time. it is cold.

Jan. 26 - I am well at this time. it is cold.

Jan. 27 - I am well at this time. it is cold.

Jan. 28, 1865 - I am well at this time. it is a very nice day.

Jan. 29 - I am well at this time. it is a nice day today.

Jan. 30 - I am well at this time. it is very cold.

Jan. 31, 1865 - I am well at this time. it is a very cold day. *[By a vote of 119 to 56, the United States House of Representatives approves the 13th Amendment to the U.S. Constitution, known as the "Anti Slavery Amendment," an important step in the legal abolition of slavery. Also see entry of February 9, 1865.]*

~ February 1865 ~

Feb. 1 - I am well at this time. it is a cold day.

Feb. 2 - I am well at this time. it is a nice day.

Feb. 3, 1865 - I am well at this time. I am going to town. *[President Lincoln holds secret meetings with Confederate Vice President Alexander Stephens in Hampton Roads, Virginia, to discuss a negotiated peace, but the effort fails.]*

Feb. 4 - I am well at this time. I am on guard.

Feb. 5 - I am well at this time. I am going to City Point. *[At Dabney's Mills and Hatcher's Run, the 142nd Pennsylvania is in action involving more than 48,350 men. Once again trying to dislodge Confederate control of key wagon supply lines leading to Petersburg, Grant launches another assault. Ephraim's friend and pen pal David Gohn is shot in the lower jaw and left hand, while seven of the color-bearers of the 142nd Pennsylvania are wounded or killed. Warren writes that Dabney's Mills, ... "was anything but a picnic." Gohn survives his wounds and after the war returns home to Jenners Cross Roads, Somerset County, where a surgeon writes of the jaw: "There is still a purulent discharge, and many pieces of bone have been extracted." (See entry of Aug. 21, 1864.)]*

Feb. 6, 1865 - I am well this mourning. I am at City Point.

Feb. 7 - I am well at this time. I am on the way to Baltimore.

Feb. 8 - I am well at this time. I just got back from City Point.

Feb. 9, 1865 - I am well at the presant time. I am on guard. *[The Commonwealth of Virginia ratifies the 13th Amendment, known as the "Anti Slavery Amendment." This vote frees 15-year-old slave Fleming Woody in Virginia. Now liberated, Woody migrates to Athens County, Ohio, where in 1891 he marries Ephraim's cousin Susanna Minerd, a legal right he did not have prior to*

Sketch of "Slaves leaving home," a scene which Ephraim's cousin by marriage, Fleming Woody—the only known slave in our extended family—may have experienced. [*Harper's Weekly*]

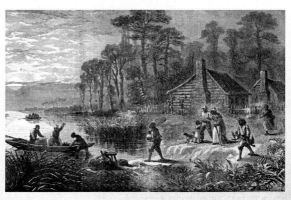

emancipation. He is the only known former slave in Ephraim's extended family.

Feb. 10 - I am well at this time. I am doing nothing.

Feb. 11 - I am well at this time. I am on guard.

Feb. 12, 1865 - I am well at the presant time. I am doing nothing.

Feb. 13 - I am well at the presant time. I am on guard to day.

Feb. 14 - I am well at the presant time. I am doing nothing to day.

Feb. 15, 1865 - I am well at the presant time. I am on guard.

Feb. 16 - I am well at the presant time. I am doing nothing.

Feb. 17 - I am well at the presant time. it is very cold.

Feb. 18, 1865 - I am well at this time. it is very cold.

Feb. 19 - I am well at this time. it is very cold. I am on guard.

Feb. 20 - I am well at this time. I am doing nothing. it is cold.

Feb. 21, 1865 - I am well at this time. I am doing nothing. it is cold.

Feb. 22 - I am well at this time. I am on guard to day.

Feb. 23 - I am well at this time. I am doing nothing to day.

Feb. 24, 1865 - I am well at this time. I am going to City Point this after noon.

Feb. 25 - I am well at this time. we are at fort monro.

Feb. 26 - I am well at this time. we are now at City Point.

Feb. 27, 1865 - I am well at this time. we are a going to leave City Point this mourning for Baltimore.

Feb. 28 - I am well at this time. We are in Camp. We got to camp at 9 oclock.

March 1865

March 1 - I am well at this time. I am doing nothing to day.

March 2, 1865 - I am well at this time. I am doing nothing to day.

March 3 - I am well at this time. I am doing nothing today. it is a nice day.

March 4 - I am well at this time. I am on guard. *[At his inauguration in Washington, D.C., Lincoln is sworn in to his second term as president.]*

March 5, 1865 - I am well at this time. I doing nothing to day. *[He leaves a word out of the last sentence.]*

March 6 - I am well at this time. I am doing nothing to day.

March 7 - I am well at this time. I am on guard.

March 8, 1865 - I am well at the presant time. I am doing nothing to day.

March 9 - I am well at this time. I am doing nothing to day.

March 10 - I am well at this time.

March 11, 1865 - I am well at this time. I am on guard to day.

March 12 - I am well at this time. I am doing nothing to day.

March 13 - I am well at this time. I am doing nothing to day.

March 14, 1865 - I am well at this time. I am on guard to day.

March 15 - I am well at this time. I am doing nothing to day.

March 16 - I am well at this time. I am doing nothing. nothing day.

March 17 1865 - I am well at the presant time. it is very cold.

March 18 - I am well at this time. I am going to Camp Bradford. I bin away for three mounts

SATURDAY 18

I am well at this time I am going to Camp Bradford I bin a way for three mounts *[months]. [After a little more than two months, the military releases Ephraim and Braun from their confinement. Ephraim returns to Camp Bradford in Baltimore.]*

March 19 - I am well at this time. I am doing nothing to day. it is very cold.

March 20, 1865 - I am well at this time. I am going to the city this morning. it is very warm.

March 21 - I am well at this time. I am on guard to day. it is very cold today.

March 22 - I am well at this time. it is very cold to day. I am going to town Washington com mence *[commence]* today.

March 23, 1865 - I am well at this time. I am on guard today. it is very cold.

March 24 - I am well at this time. I am going to town today. it is very cold.

March 25 - I am well at this time. I am on guard today. camp guard. it is cold and cloudey.

March 26, 1865 - Camp Bradford Baltimore - I am well at this time. it is very cold this mourning. I am doing nothing to day.

March 27 - I am well at this time. I am on guard to day. it is a nice day.

March 28 - I am well at this time. I am going to the city this day. it is a very nice day. *[The 142nd Pennsylvania is part of the Appomattox Campaign as the war nears its end. At the Lewis Farm near Gravelly Run, Union forces make another attack on the Boydton Plank Road and the South Side Railroad. Writes Warren: "The enemy in our front were pouring in a tremendous shower of bullets; I ordered the men to lie down and commence firing as fast as ever they could, which they did. Their firing being low was very effective, for in our immediate front we were holding them, and giving them more than they wished for. We are not very far from Five Forks and the South Side Road, and I was in great hopes that before night we should have it."]*

March 29, 1865 - Camp Bradford Baltimore - I am well at this time I am on guard to day it is a very nice day

March 30 - I am not very well. I haf a very bad cold. it is raining this mourning. it is very wet this mourning. I am doing nothing today.

March 31 - I am well at this time. I am on guard to day. it is a going to raine. it is very mudy. [*At White Oak Road, the 142nd Pennsylvania is among Union troops entrenched along the Boydton Plank Road facing an enemy led by Major General Bushrod R. Johnson. Meanwhile, Union Major General Philip H. Sheridan, attempting to finally destroy the South Side Railroad, is blocked by Confederate cavalry under Major General George E. Pickett.*]

~ *April 1865* ~

April 1, 1865 - Camp Bradford Baltimore - I am well at this time. I am doing nothing. I am going to town this after noon it is a very nice day. [*The 142nd Pennsylvania fights at Five Forks, an intersection of roads considered as the most critical along the entire Petersburg front. Cavalry under Sheridan and Pickett jockey to determine who will finally control the South Side Railroad. Lee tells Confederate President Jefferson Davis that Petersburg and Richmond must be evacuated. Warren writes: "The next morning our forces advanced and took the South-side Railroad, Five Forks, and about 13,000 prisoners. This broke the enemy all up, and General Lee immediately thereafter withdrew from Petersburg and tried hard to make good his escape, which he failed to do, so closely was he pursued… Five Forks was the last hard-fought battle of the war."*]

Union army enters the long-sought Petersburg, following a nine-month siege of trench warfare. [*Harper's Weekly*, April 22, 1865]

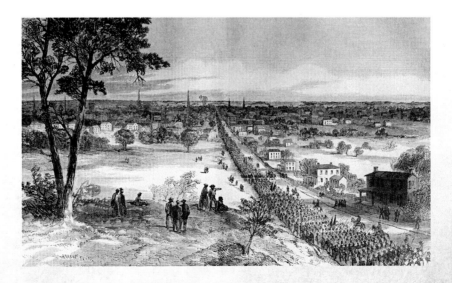

April 2 - I am well at presant time. I am doing nothing only going on dress perraid *[parade]* at 4 o'clock this eavening. it is a nice day. *[Confederate government officials flee Richmond.]*

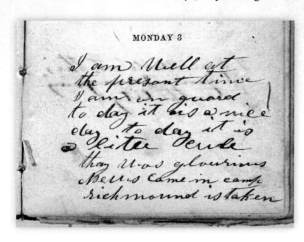

MONDAY 3

April 3 - I am well at the presant time. I am on guard to day. it is a nice day today. it is a litle cule *[little cool]*. they was glourious news come in camp. richmound is taken. *[At long last, the prize of the Confederacy, its capitol city, comes under Union control. Fleeing Southern troops burn bridges and warehouses to prevent their capture, and the flames turn into a larger conflagration destroying about one quarter of the city.]*

Having captured the Confederate capital of Richmond, the victorious Union army streams into the city. *[Harper's Weekly, April 22, 1865]*

April, 4 1865 - Camp Bradford Baltimore - I am well at the present. I am doing nothing today. it is a nice day. good news from the army of the potomack.

April 5 - I am well at this time.

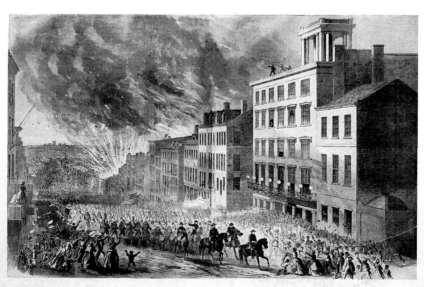

I am guard to day. it is a very nice day.

April 6 - I am well at this time. I am going to the city.

April 7, 1865 - Camp Baltimore - I am well at this time. I am on guard to day. *[Ephraim's cousin by marriage, William J. Burditt, is shot in the thigh after being captured by Confederate forces in Farmville, Virginia. (See entry of July 14, 1864.)]*

April 8 - I am well at this time. I am doing nothing today. it is a nice day.

April 9 - I am well at this time. I am on guard to day. *[With his army fleeing, but collapsing at Appomattox Court House after making one final attempt to fight, Lee surrenders. The 142nd Penn-sylvania is stationed at Appomattox and escorts captured stores to Burkesville Station. Warren writes that Lee was: "so completely hemmed in and surrounded that sooner than see the useless waste of the lives of his brave army he sent to our lines a flag of truce. And soon the news of his surrender was heralded to the world." The surrender is signed later that day, in a face to face meeting between Lee and Grant in the parlor of a private home. Major George Armstrong Custer is among the officers attending the ceremony. In a twist of fate, Custer's younger brother, Capt. Thomas Ward Custer, recipient of two Medals of Honor, produc-es a child out of wedlock six years later with Ephraim's cousin Rebecca Minerd, of Tontogany, Ohio.]*

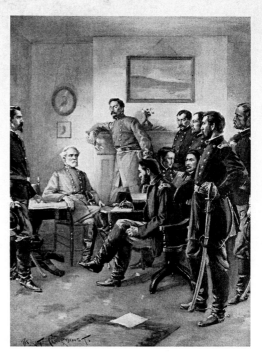

Gen. Lee surrenders to Gen. Grant at Appomattox, Va. Among the observers is Gen. George Armstrong Custer, at far right. [*The Century Magazine*]

April 10, 1865 - Camp Bradford Baltimore - I am well at the presant time. I am going to city point this after noon. it is raining.

April 11 - I am well at the present time. We are at fortes monroe this mourning. we are going to start for city point at 10 o'clock.

April 12 - I am well at this time. we are at city point. We are agoing to leave for baltimore.

April 13, 1865 - Camp Bradford Baltimore - I am well at this time. We just got back from city point. it is raining.

April 14 - I am well at this time. I am going to drill to day. it is a very nice day. *[While attending a performance of "Our American Cousin" at Ford's Theatre in Washington, D.C., President Lincoln is shot by John Wilkes Booth, and dies the next morning in a rooming house across the street.]*

April 15 - I am well at this time. I am going to town. there is very bad news. old president lincoln is kild. it is to bad *[too bad]*.

April 16, 1865 - Camp Bradford Baltimore - I am well at the present time. I am on guard today. it is a very nice day. I wood like to be in old turkey foot to day. *[Shocked by the irony and senselessness of Lincoln's murder, Ephraim likely is eager to share in mourning the loss and sharing opinions with his grandfather Yankee John Younkin and family back home.]*

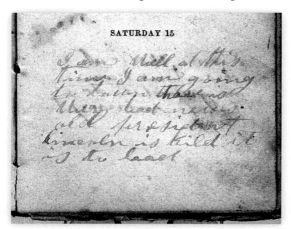

April 17 - I am well at this time. I am drilling to day. it is a very nice day.

April 18 - I am well at this time. I am on guard to day. it is raining today.

April 19, 1865 - Camp Bradford Baltimore - I am well at this time. I am doing nothing today. it is a very nice day. it very warm. there is grait deal of firing today. president furneal. *[Ephraim refers to Lincoln's funeral procession in Washington. D.C., where* the coffin is escorted down Pennsylvania Avenue from the White House to the rotunda of the Capitol Building, accompanied by the sound of firing guns and tolling church bells.]

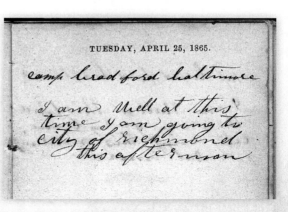

WEDNESDAY, APRIL 19, 1865.

April 20 - I am well at this time. I am going to drill this after noon. it is a going to rain. it is very warm this mourning.

April 21 - I am well at this time. I am on guard to day. it is very wet thos few days. [Lincoln's funeral car travels by rail from Washington, D.C. to Baltimore, with members of the VRC serving as guards. Whether Ephraim sees any of the funeral procession or hearse car is unknown.]

April 22, 1865 - Camp Bradford Baltimore - I am well at the present time. I am doing nothing to day. it is a very nice day.

April 23 - I am well at this time. I am on guard to day. it is very cold. most cold a mong to [illegible].

April 24 - I am well at this time. I am doing nothing to day. I just got off guard. it is cule [cool].

April 26, 1865 - Camp Bradford Baltimore - I am well at this time. I am going to city of Richmond this afternoon. [With Richmond as the highly sought prize during the war, imagine what Ephraim would have seen, thought and felt upon entering the former Confederate capitol city. The same day, President Lincoln's assassin Booth is shot and killed in a burning Virginia tobacco barn.]

TUESDAY, APRIL 25, 1865.

April 26 - I am well at this time. we are at fort Monroe. we are now at new port news. it is one o'clock.

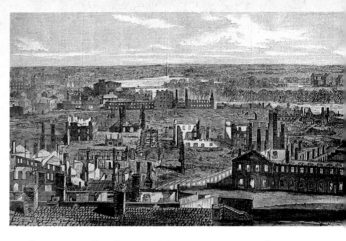

Ruins of Richmond, which Ephraim would have seen in late April 1865 [*Harper's Weekly*, June 17, 1865]

April 27 - I am well at this time. We are at city point at the present time. We are a going to Peters burg this afternoon. I am now in Peters Burgh, siting in the Market hous [*sitting in the market house*]. We are a going to leave this evening.

April 28, 1865 - Camp Bradford Baltimore - I am well at this time. We are a going leave city point this mourning for baltimore.

April 29 - I am well at this time. We are now in Washington city. We are a going to leave fort baltimore this eavening at fore o'clock.

April 30 - I am not very well this mourning. We are a going to be musterd for pay at 10 o'clock. it is a very nice day.

~ *May 1865* ~

May 1, 1865 - Camp bradford baltimore - I am not well at this time. it is raining this mourning.

May 2 - I am not eney better this mourning. it is a very nice day.

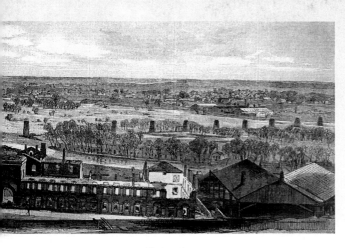

May 3 - I am not eney better yet.

May 4, 1865 - Camp bradford baltimore - I am a good deale beter this mourning. it is a very nice day. it is very plesant this mourning. [*After a funeral of 19 days with public viewings in 13 cities, and passing through seven states, Lincoln's remains are laid to rest in Springfield, Illinois.*]

May 5 - I am nearly well this mourning. I am getting beter fast. I took a walk out in the country yesterday. every thing looks so plesant in the country. I wold lik too be at home.

May 6 - I am well at this time. I am detaled too work in the couch hous [*coach house?*] today. it rained very hard last knight.

May 7, 1865 - Camp bradford baltimore - I am well at the present. I am on guard to day. it is very warm.

WEDNESDAY 3

I am not eney beter yet

FRIDAY 5

I am nearley Well this mourning I am giting beter fast I took a Walk out in the country yester day every thing looks so plesant in the country I wold tik too be at home

May 8 - I am well at this time. I am doing nothing too day. it is very hot.

May 9 - I am well at this time. I am doing nothing too day. it is raining too day.

May 10, 1865 - camp bradford baltimore - I am well at this time. I am doing nothing too day. it is cloudy too day. we have very good times hear at the presant time. I think we will have good times til our time is out.

May 11, 1865 - camp bradford baltimore - I am well at this time. I am doing nothing to day. it is a very nice day this fore mourn but it lookes for raine. and oful [an awful] storm coming up this after noon.

May 12 - I am well at this time. it is very windy. it rained very hard last knight.

May 13, 1865 - camp bradford baltimore - I am well at the presant time. I am scroubeing [scrubbing] our barracks to day. it is a very nice day to day.

May 14 - I am well at this time. I am doing nothing. I am a going to take a walk out in the country.

May 15 - I am well at this time. I am doing nothing to day. it is a very nice day.

May 16, 1865 - camp bradford baltimore - I am well at this time. I am on guard to day. it is very hot. we are under marching orders to go to penna.

THURSDAY 18

May 17 - I am well at this time. I am doing nothing to day. it is very hot. we are expected to go away every day. I am going to the city this eavening.

May 18 - I am well at this time. I am doing nothing today. it is very hot. we are not going a way from this camp yet a while. I think we will stay at this camp until our time is out.

May 19, 1865 - camp bradford baltimore - I am well at this time. I am doing nothing. it rained very hard last knight.

May 20 - I am well at this time. I am doing nothing to day. it is a very hot.

May 21 - I am well at this time. I am doing nothing. it is very [?] this few dayes. [Ephraim leaves a word out of the last sentence.]

May 22, 1865 - camp bradford baltimore - I am well at this time. we got mourning orders last night. we are a going leave at fore o'clock this after noon. we are going to cloumbus [Columbus] ohio.

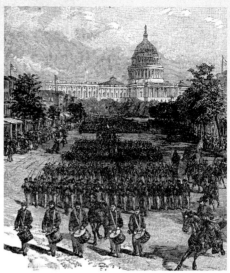

May 23 - I am well at this time. we are in harrisbourgh [Harrisburg, Pennsylvania]. we are a going to leave at 8 oclock. [The 142nd Pennsylvania marches in the Grand Review before President Andrew Johnson in Washington. Walt Whitman, watching on Pennsylvania Avenue, writes to his mother: "Imagine a great wide avenue like Flatbush avenue [with] solid ranks of soldiers… just marching steady all day long for two days… "]

Soldiers of the 142nd Pennsylvania, among 100,000 Union troops, march in the Grand Review in Washington, D.C. before President Andrew Johnson on May 24, 1865.

May 24 - I am well at this time. we are in ohio.

May 25, 1865 - Ohio - Soldiers home columbous - I am well at this time. we are in cloumbus ohio at souldiers home. we are doing nothing. it is very wet at presant time. [The soldiers' home, previously known as Tripler Hospital in Columbus, and located near Camp Chase, is used to provide medical care for sick soldiers at Chase. After the war, the federal government donates the home to the state of Ohio. The facility later is re-established in Dayton, Ohio.]

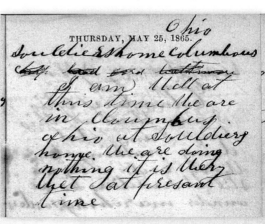

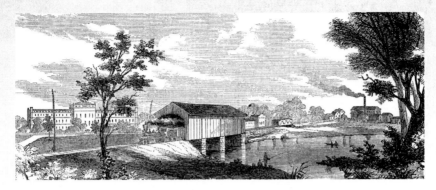

Railroad through Columbus, from a sketch before the war. [1857 newspaper]

May 26 - I am well at this time. I am stil doing nothing. we are stil at souldiers home at columbous Ohio. it rained very hard last knight.

May 27 - I am well at this time. I am stil doing nothing. we are stil at souldiers home, columbous Ohio.

May 28, 1865 - Camp tod Columbous Ohio - I am well at this time. I am stil doing nothing. it is very cule. we are stil at souldiers home under marching orders.

May 29 - Camp tod Columbus Ohio - I am well at this time. I am doing nothing only drill a little. it is very warm to day. we are a going to leave this eavening. [*The 142nd Pennsylvania officially musters out of military service.*]

May 30 - Camp denson Ohio - I am well at this time. we got to this camp this mourning. it is very nice plas. we have very hard times. [*Camp Dennison is Ephraim's final stop in the war, located 16 miles from Cincinnati, with VRC soldiers serving there as hospital guards. Ephraim's comments about "very hard times" may have to do with lack of supplies or the poor quality of food. In Ohio in the War Whitelaw Reid states: "Through the autumn of 1864 complaints as to the food of patients at Camp Dennison were rife—particularly complaints as to the food of convalescents." An investigation by C.S. Tripler, the Army's medical director in Cincinnati, leads to "harsh judgment" of the camp leadership for "mistreatment of the soldiers" including "insufficient and deteriorated food." The matter comes to the attention of Ohio Governor John Brough, who becomes frustrated with the intellectual arrogance of the camp's physician leadership, and writes: "Still no remedy was proposed; no change of officials recommended; no remedy for the wrongs or sufferings of our men pointed out; but the scarred and wounded veterans of a score of battle-fields*]

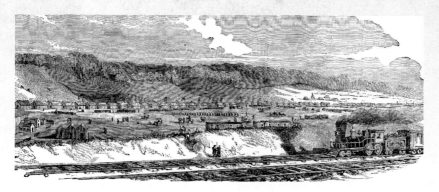

were coolly sacrificed to the esprit de corps of the medical profession." When Ephraim later tells his grandchildren of being so hungry that he would have eaten muddy meat, he may well have been referring to his experience at Dennison.]

Sprawling Camp Dennison, Ohio, where Ephraim's wartime service ended. [*Famous Leaders and Battle Scenes of the Civil War*]

May 31, 1865 - Camp denson Ohio - I am well at this time. we had a mounthely inspection today. it is very hot.

~ June 1865 ~

June 1 - I am well at this time. I am doing nothing. it is thankes giving day today. [*In response to Lincoln's assassination, June 1, 1865 is proclaimed a national day of fasting and prayer. There is precedence to this holiday, as Lincoln himself declared two national days of thanksgiving, first on Aug. 6, 1863 after the army's victory at Gettysburg, and on Nov. 26, 1863, coinciding with harvest celebrations all across the northern states.]*

June 2 - I am well at this time. I am doing nothing to day. it is very warm.

June 3, 1865 - Camp Denison Ohio - Cincinanati - I am well at this time. I am white washing today. it is very warm.

June 4 - I am well at this time. I am going on in specting this mourning. it is very hot.

June 5 - I am well at this time. I am white washing to day. it is very hot and dri.

THURSDAY, JUNE 1

I am well at this time I am doing nothing it is thankes giving day to day

June 6, 1865 - Camp Dennison Ohio - Cincinnati - I am well at this time. I am white washing to day. it is very hot.

June 7 - I am well at this time. I am white washing to day. it is very hot.

June 8 - I am well at this time. I am doing nothing to day. it is very hot and dry.

June 9, 1865 - Camp Dennison Ohio Near Cincinnati - I am well at this time. I am doing nothing this day. it is very hot. we had a heave raine last knight.

June 10 - I am well at this time. I am doing nothing to day. it is very hot.

June 11 - I am well at the present time. I am on for tig *[fatigue duty?]*. it is very warm this day.

June 12, 1865 - Camp Dennison Near Cincinatti Ohio - I am well at this time. I am doing nothing.

June 13 - I am well at this time. I am on for tig [?] today. it lookes for raine.

Religious services at Camp Dennison, Ohio. [*Harper's Weekly*, June 1861]

June 14 - I am well at this time. I am doing nothing today. it is very hot.

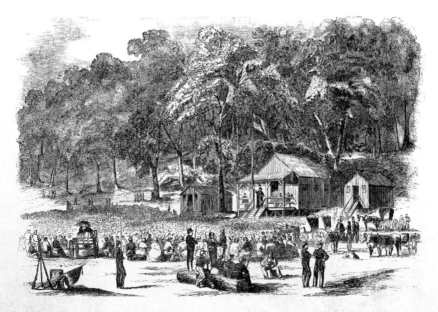

June 15, 1865 - Camp Dennison Near Cincinatti Ohio - I am well at this time. I am doing nothing. it is very warm and dry.

June 16 - I am well at this time. I am on for tig to day. it rained very hard.

June 17 - I am well at this time. I am doing nothing to day. it is very warm.

June 18, 1865 - Camp Dennison Ohio Near Cincinnati - I am well at this time. I am doing nothing to day. it is very warm.

June 19 - I am well at this time. I am on guard to day.

June 20 - I am well at this time. I am doing nothing to day. it s very warm.

June 21, 1865 - Camp Dennison near Cincinnati Ohio - I am well at this time. I am doing nothing today. it is very warm.

June 22 - I am well at this time. I am on guard today. it is very warm.

June 23 - I am well at this time. I am doing nothing today. it is warm.

June 24, 1865 - Camp Dennison Ohio - I am well at this time. I am on guard to day. it is very hot.

June 25 - I am well at this time. I am doing nothing to day. it is very warm.

June 26 - I am well at this time. I am doing nothing to day. it rained very hard last knight.

June 27, 1865 - Camp Dennison Ohio Near Cincinnati - I am well at this time. I am on guard to day. it is very cule this mourning.

June 28 - I am well at this time. I am doing nothing to day. it is very warm today.

June 29 - I am well at this time. I am doing nothing to day. it is very warm.

June 30, 1865 - Camp Dennison Ohio - I am well at this time. I am on guard to day. we got mousterd in for pay the last day of June.

~ July 1865 ~

July 1 - I am well at this time. I was mustard out of the unite state sourvours [United States service] this after noon.

July 2 - I am well at this time. it is very warm.

July 3, 1865 - Camp Dennison Ohio - I am well at this time. I am stil in camp Dennison.

July 4 - I am well at this time. I am going to Cincinnati to tak my fourth ["Take my Fourth"—participation in a Fourth of July celebration]. I just got back from town. thare was a grate time thare.

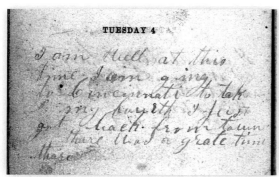

July 5 - I am well at this time. we was to get our pay to day but we wont get pay til tomourow.

July 6, 1865 - Camp Dennison, Ohio - I am well at this. I am in green county at present time. [Having received his final pay, Ephraim makes the rail trip from Cincinnati to near Jacktown, Greene County, Pennsylvania, to see his parents and siblings. Ephraim's parents have been living in Greene County for several years. His sisters Susan (Birch), Nancy (Farabee) and Catherine (Bedillion) and brothers Andrew, Henry Harrison and Elias also reside in the area. Having viewed some of the most grisly head and facial wounds imaginable during the war, one can only imagine Ephraim's emotions when gazing again into the scarred eyes and face of his 51-year-old mother, who has never recovered from her burns. The reunion reaction of Ephraim to his strong-willed father, who earlier objected so strenuously to his sons' enlistment, is unknown. At about this time, Ephraim's brother Chance is living in Zanesville, Ohio, never to return home, and eventually migrates to Illinois. Among other news Ephraim likely learns during his return is of his *sister Susan's courtship with widowed Civil War veteran Samuel Birch, who served with the 16th Pennsylvania Cavalry which distinguished itself at Gettysburg.]*

July 7 - I am well at this time. I am at my old father.

July 8 - ratle route spice sasfrass while chery bark hant full of each in one gallon water boil.

July 9, 1865 - from jacksonville to wanes bourgh *[Waynesburg]* 6 miles from wanes bourgh to jefferson 8 miles and from jefferson to the river 3 miles from the rier

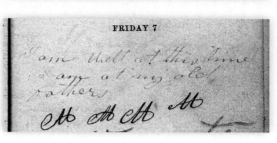

to surights 85 miles and from thare to counelsville. *[Connellsville]* 13 miles from Counelsville to spring field *[Springfield, later renamed Normalville]* 8 miles. *[Here, Ephraim records the details of his travel from his parents' home in Greene County to*

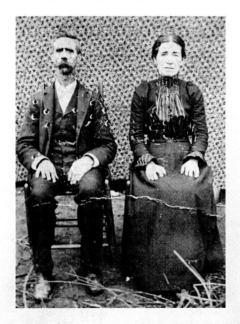

Left: Ephraim's sister and brother in law, Nancy and Spencer Farabee, to whom Ephraim immediately went to see upon his discharge, in Greene County, Pennsylvania.

Below: Ephraim's father Henry Minerd.

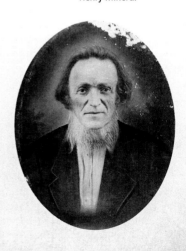

his permanent home in Somerset County. He repeats these notes in his entry of July 12, adding the final leg of his trip from Springfield to Kingwood.]

July 10 - *[blank]*

July 11 - thare is a big meeting at the stone meeting house ending crick on the 9 of June.

WEDNESDAY, JULY 12, 1865.

from jacksonville to Wanes burgh 16 miles from Wanes the burgh to jefferson 8 miles and from jefferson to the River 3 miles from the river to See wright 85 miles and thare to Counels ville 13 miles from Counels ville

THURSDAY 13

to Springfield 9 miles

from Springfield to King Wood 9 miles

62

July 12, 1865 - from jacksonville to wanes burgh 16 miles from wanes burgh to jefferson 8 miles and from jefferson to the river 3 miles from the river to see wright 85 miles and thare to Conels ville to Springfield 9 miles from spring filed to king wood 9 miles 62.

July 15 - When you see this remember me. the merry smiles a part we bee. We haf to be content *[with]* it the best we can with pen and ink.

July 21 - beenes and peese, wheat and potato and corn punkin seads, Andrew Shrock one day thrashing. one half day gathring shuger watter. one day pealing bark. one day cleding *[clearing?]* trees. one day helpting at the barne. Wone day thrashing work in harvest July16 1866. wone day three days and a half cradling and one day and three quarters moing *[mowing]*. *[No longer needing a diary to record his war travels, Ephraim converts its usage into a commonplace book filled with notes about his labors, wages and events.]*

July 24 - David Schrock. Wone day sprouting / wone day sprouting / wone day grubing / one half day grubing / half day houling doung IIIIII *[tally marks]*. wone half day houling doung. Wone day hauling Stone. wone half day moing. wone half day moing. wone half day pitching hay. wone day moing. wone day moing. wone day moing. three quartes of a day

moing. five days and half in harvest. five days in the spring.
[Some of these entries have tally marks beside them.]

July 19 *[repeated July 27]* - What a pleasure it is for to have a
good wife Now one who is able and willing to cheer and to
comfort a man through his life. one who knows how to eke
out a shilling of my own little wife. I can't grumble at all, but
my familys run enough rather thirteen boys and girls. I have
got great and small and that's a nice sight for a father.

July 30 - There's anna maria a young woman grown the lord
knows. I wish she would marry. She goes out every night .
I can't keep her at home with a young chap who calls
himself harry.

~ August 1865 ~

Aug. 1 - Edward harnet *[Harned?]* three dolars albert andrews
four dolars

Aug. 8, 1865 - one half day cradeling. fred Kreager wone half
day binding oats.

Aug. 9 1865 - Joannah Miner. days and years are loung.

Aug. 11, 1865 - Andrew S. work in harest *[harvest]*. July
the 16 1866. three days and a half cradeling. One day and a
half moing.

Aug. 12 - Done six days moing. the seond weak third weak
four days tenn days moing.

~ September 1865 ~
the towns in the war

Harrous Burg
[Harrisburg], Penna

Baltimore MD.

Washington City DC

Fredrick City MD

West Middle town MD

Boomes Bour *[Boonsboro]* MD

Sharps Burgh MD

Burlinn *[Berlin]* MD

Worington
[Warrington] VA

Fredrick Burgh
[Fredericksburg] VA

Alexandria VA

Philadelpia [Philadelphia] Penna

New Jursey City

New Yourk City

Albaney City NY

Buflow City NY

Youcut [Utica] NY

Cleaven land [Cleveland] Penna [sic]

Cloumbus Ohio

Indinaples [Indianapolis] India [Indiana]

Michigan City India

fourtos monro [Fortress Monroe]

City point Va

Peters Burgh Va

Johnstown Penna

Altonah Penna

Pitts Burgh Penna

Cincinnatia ohio

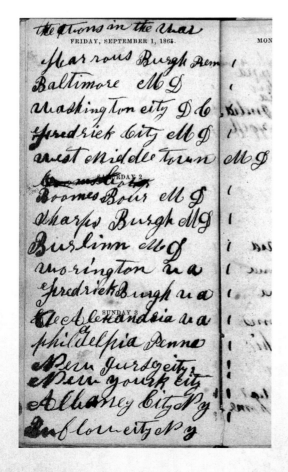

the End of my Journey in the War. Now in peace at home.

[Ephraim records all the places he saw during the war.]

Sept. 8 - September washing for me Elisabeth Andrews. [Details about Andrews are not known.]

~ October 1865 ~

Oct. 7, 1865 - hourse in pasture at William. Ephraim Miner. [signs his own name]

Oct. 10, 1865 - Moses King 50 [cents]. J. Dumbauld 100 50. Christfor Kreager 50. Andrews 37 cents.

Oct. 13, 1865 - Work for Harmond Younkin November the first one day. [Harmon "Herman" Younkin, a cousin, becomes Ephraim's father in law the year after the war. Harman is well known as a farmer and Methodist preacher in Turkeyfoot Township. Both Ephraim and Harmon are mentioned in a chapter about Harman's son, John F. Younkin, in the 1899 book, Biographical Review Containing Life Sketches of Leading Citizens of Bedford and Somerset Counties.]

Oct. 14 - Wone day choping slead [?] trees. Wone day hauling bourdes [boards].

~ *November 1865* ~

Nov. 12 - Saturday the 8. Ephraim Miner Ephra Ephraim Ephraim Minerd [doodles his signature, using varying spellings of the family name]

Nov. 24, 1865 - I am well at this time. I am at home this mourning at papes [Papa's]. [Having visited his parents in early July 1865, he returns to Greene County to see them again.]

Nov. 27, 1865 - I am well at this time. I am at my sisters, Nancys. it is very cole and chilley. [At this time, Ephraim's beloved sister Nancy is age 17, has been married for three years to Spencer Farabee, and resides near her parents in Greene County. Ephraim and Nancy continue to visit each other

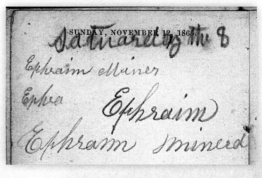

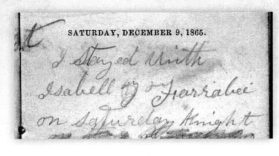

SATURDAY, DECEMBER 9, 1865.

I stayed with Isabell & Farrabee on Saturday Knight

for the remaining 50 years of their lives.

Nov. 29 - I am well at this time it is very cold.

~ December 1865 ~

Dec. 4, 1865 - I stayed with Isabell Farrabee on Mounday knight. *[Isabell Farabee is a sister of Ephraim's brother-in-law Spencer Farabee and resides in Greene County. She is age 16 and either is, or is about to become, the bride of carpenter William Pettit.]*

Dec. 8 - I am at my sisters Nanecy.

Dec. 9, 1865 - I stayed with Isabell Farrabee on Saturday Knight.

Dec. 24, 1865 - Moses King 50 cents. Cristefort Kreager 50. Andrew Schrock too days and half. David Schroeck 4 days and a half. *[King and Kreager apparently are Ephraim's friends, Andrew Schrock is Ephraim's uncle, and David Schrock's connection is not yet known.]*

Ephraim's uncle and aunt, Charles and Adaline (Harbaugh) Minerd, into whose home he moved in January 1866.

~ 1866 ~

I moved to Charley Miners on January the second 1866. *[Charles and Adaline (Harbaugh) Minerd are Ephraim's uncle and aunt, and are cousins who had married each other. They live in the old Minerd homeplace in the hollow below the Old Bethel Church of God. Ephraim spends the winter here and gets to know the Minerd children—Lucinda J. (age 16), Rebecca "Jennie" (age 14), Josephine (age 12), Martha Emma "Matt" (age 9), Lawson (age 7), Almira Malissa (age 3) and Grant (age 1, apparently named after the famous Union general). Heartache rocks the family on March 10, 1866, when the black-haired, black-eyed infant Grant dies of the croup. Ephraim's lodgings there are only temporary, as the following year, the Minerds move to a 290-acre farm at Maple Summit, along the "old Turkeyfoot road" in nearby Fayette County.]*

Thursday 8 - Moved to Charley Miner. January the 2 1866. on day thrashing rhy. one day thrashing oats. a hanker chief. washing at Charley. paid up to the april the 2, 1866. [*Ephraim's timekeeping notes recording his labors.*]

I got married on the 28th of October 1866. [*Ephraim's bride, Joanna Younkin, is the daughter of Herman and Susan (Faidley) Younkin. This is the third consecutive generation of marriages between Minerd men and Younkin women. He makes no other mention of the wedding and writes this in an available blank space in the diary, in the space for Aug. 20, 1865.*]

~ *Memoranda* ~
[*in the back of the 1865 diary*]

J. Durling 80 dolars

F. stackweather 25

Nelson sharp one dolar. [*Nelson Sharp, Ephraim's fellow member of the 22nd VRC. See more on Sharp in the section of this book entitled "Ephraim's Friends."*]

Ephraim Miner is my name. Single is my life. hapy shall the girl be who gives me my wife.

PART VI

Ephraim's Friends

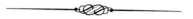

Letter Writing Correspondents

[Note—the following names appear in the back of 1865 diary, representing letters Ephraim receives that year. This suggests he was an active correspondent, even though none of his letters to family and friends back home has been found.]

Mifs Nelly Mulcahy, Cohoes P.o. Albany NY IIII II
[Ephraim apparently befriends Mulcahy while in Albany, and writes her name and address on several pages of the diary.]

Mifs Joannha Younkin IIII III

Mifs Martha Reem IIII II

Juley litle 160 Webb St bet mill and stone *[between Mill and Stone]*

Fredrick Dumbauld 13 dolars

Kuntee 12 dolars

h. walter 15 dolars

Rush one dolar

Isabell Farbee IIII *[Sister in law of Ephraim's married sister Nancy Farabee]*

Mifs Mary ann Dumbauld IIII IIII IIII IIII IIII III

Mifs Susan Younkin IIII IIII IIII II *[Ephraim's cousin]*

Mifs Christeane Dumbauld IIII IIII

Mifs Joann Miner IIII IIII IIII IIII I *[Ephraim's first cousin, and sister of Martin Miner]*

Mifs Louisa kreager IIII IIII IIII IIII

Miss Caroline Schrock IIII II

Peter Dumbauld III

Andrew Schrock IIII *[Ephraim's uncle by marriage]*

Eli Miner IIII IIII *["Eli" may refer to Ephraim's younger brother Elias Minor, age 12, but more likely to his uncle, Eli Minerd, age 34, known to be literate and only eight years older than Ephraim.]*

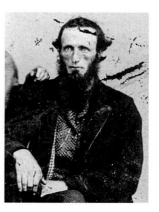

Eli Minerd,
Ephriam's uncle

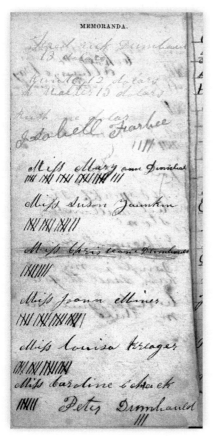

Solmon Rugh IIII IIII III

phil cutshall IIII

David gohn IIII IIII

Benjimmon lohr IIII

John hoover III

David Kifer IIII

george thomas IIII

M. firestone IIII

jacob pritts IIII

John Trimpey III

Signatures in the Diary

[Note—the following signatures appear in the back of 1865 diary, a group of fellow soldiers Ephraim befriends during the war, primarily members of the 22nd VRC.]

C.W. Newcomb, Pittstown, Rensselear Co., NY *[Cyrenus W. Newcomb, 2nd New York Infantry and 169th New York Infantry—He stands 5 feet, 10 inches tall. Enlisting in 1861, he becomes sick and is treated in the hospital at Fortress Monroe. Discharged from the army at Newport News, Virginia, at year's end, he re-enlists in the 169th New York Infantry in August 1862. While on duty at White House Landing, Virginia, in 1863, he suffers from rheumatism and hemorrhoids, and is* treated at Balfour Hospital in Portsmouth, Virginia. Later, he transfers to the 22nd VRC, where he meets Ephraim. After the war, he resides in Pittstown, Brunswick and Poestenkill, New York, where he earns a small living as a shoemaker in a country store. Physicians treat him for heart disease and buildup of fluids. A friend notes "when sitting down he seemed in misery [and] it seemed to hurt him to sit square on a seat, would sit leaning to one side." He dies on Dec. 8, 1903.]

Wesley Long, East Hamburg, Erie Co., NY [116th Regiment, New York Infantry— He stands 5 feet, 4 inches tall and is a merchant before the war. While on duty at Baltimore in 1862, he contracts fever while sleeping on the ground during heavy rains, leading to kidney and throat problems. He is treated at Chesapeake Hospital at Fortress Monroe and transfers to the 22nd VRC in August 1863. He is assigned to Camp Dennison, Ohio, where he meets Ephraim, and is there at war's end. He settles in Cardington, Ohio, where he is a harness maker and may have known Ephraim's cousins Elizabeth (Minor) Wilson Armstrong and Margaret (Miner) Sloan Maxwell. Wesley marries Sarah Wolfe in 1867, and they have two children, Hubert and Edith. In 1891, surgeons note his disease of kidneys and throat and his "haggard appearance." Wesley dies on Jan. 17, 1893.]

Marion Jackson, Dresden, Muskingum Co, Ohio [Pvt, 122nd Regiment, Ohio Infantry]

Peter V. Orcutt, West Fort, Ann Washington Co NY [169th Regiment, New York Infantry; 22nd Regiment, VRC]

John W. Gilliland, Boonsboro, Boone Co, Iowa [32nd Iowa Infantry]

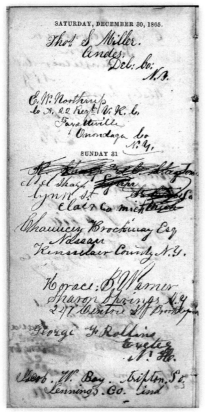

Thos. S. Miller, Andes, Del. Co., NY

E.W. Northrup, Co. A, 22 Reg't, V.R.C.,
Fayetteville, Onondaga Co., NY

N. Sharp, Lynn St., Clair Co., Mich.
*[Nelson Oscar Sharp, 5th Michigan Cavalry.
At the battle of Williamsport in July 1863,
he suffers a hernia while jumping his horse
over a wall, landing hard on the saddle horn.
He is treated at Warrington Junction, Virginia, and at Lincoln Hospital in Washington,
D.C., where he meets Ephraim. Both are
transferred to the VRC in July 1864 and
remain together until the end of the war.
Ephraim views the rupture more than once,
including when they swim in the Little Miami
River at Camp Dennison in July 1865. After
the war, he lives in Lynn, Michigan, and in
1866 marries Hannah Elizabeth Richardson. They have four children: Albert E.,
Nelson, Martha and William Sharp. They
divorce in 1882, and he marries widow Nellie (Reid) Montgomery. In 1899, Ephraim
writes affidavits in support of Sharp's claim
for a military pension. He dies of uremic poisoning at Reno City, Michigan, on Oct. 3, 1918, at the age of 73.]*

Chauncey Brockway Esq., Nassau, Rensselear Co., NY
*[169th New York Infantry—Standing 5 feet, 5 inches tall,
Chauncey Griffith Brockway endures "nervous prostration"
and shortness of breath caused by "over-exertion" while on a
march from White House Landing to Fortress Monroe in 1863.
Treated at Balfour General Hospital in Portsmouth, Virginia,
he is transferred to the 22nd VRC and is discharged from the
army at Camp Dennison in 1865. He never marries, and
spends the rest of his years farming in Nassau, suffering from
heart disease. Later in life, a friend observes, he has "no back
teeth and not a whole one in front." He dies on or about May
22, 1899.]*

Horace B. Warner, Sharon Springs, N.Y., 247 Centre St., Brooklyn *[22nd New York Infantry National Guard (30 days) and 7th New York Heavy Artillery]*

George F. Rollins, Exeter, N.H. *[13th New Hampshire Infantry —At Newport News, Virginia, in March 1863, he suffers chills, fever and malaria. Treated in military hospitals in Suffolk and Petersburg, Virginia, he transfers to the VRC in September 1863, where he meets Ephraim at Camp Dennison. After the war, he returns home to Exeter, New Hampshire. He marries Clara J. Moulton in 1867, producing two children, Fred and Nellie Rollins. George is a brick mason but claims to have lost about three-quarters of his ability to earn a living because of his wartime disability. In later years, unable to perform manual labor, all he can do is take "care of a small garden and doing chores around home. He is confined to the house four or five days at a time, as often as once in three or four weeks…," says a friend. He dies at the age of 46 on April 5, 1890.]*

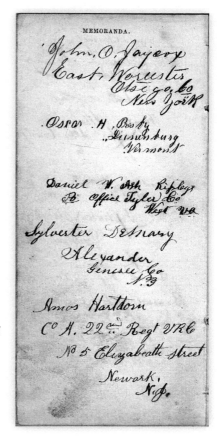

Jacob W. Bay, Tripton P.O., Jennings Co., ind. *[89th Indiana Infantry, 22nd Indiana Infantry, 52nd Indiana Infantry]*

John C. Jaycox, East Corcester, Otsego Co, NY *[121st New York Infantry]*

Oscar H. Presly, Lunenburg, Vermont

Daniel W. Ash, Ripley Po Office, Tyler Co., West Va. *[10th West Virginia Infantry —Enlisting in 1864 at Wheeling, West Virginia, he stands 6 feet tall. In battle at Winchester, Virginia, in 1864, he is hit in the upper back, with the musket ball passing near his spine and lodging near his right scapula, where surgeons cut it out. He is soon after transferred to the 22nd VRC. After the war, he resides in Centreville and Sancho, Tyler County, West Virginia. He*

Actual surgeon's sketch of Daniel Ash's gunshot wound.
[National Archives]

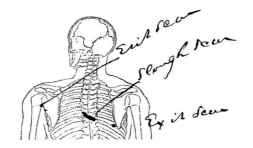

marries Nancy K. Smith in 1867, and they have three children: Anna Della, Theodicia and Nina Ash. After Nancy dies in 1877, he marries again, to Rebecca Woodburn, in 1879, and they have three more children: Otto Daniel, Alice M. and Irvin Odie Ash. Suffering from lung problems caused by his wound, Daniel passes away on Feb. 21, 1888.]

Sylvester DeMary, Alexander, Genesee Co., NY [2nd New York Heavy Artillery and 9th New York Heavy Artillery—A decade before the war breaks out, he marries Arvilla in Attica, New York He stands 5 feet, 8 inches tall. While at Fort Simmons in Washington, D.C., he suffers a hernia when installing heavy timbers on a gun bed for a 1,000 lb. cannon. Then, in the battle of Cedar Creek, Virginia, in 1864, he is shot in the left hand, with the ball exiting through the palm, severing tendons. Transferred to the 22nd VRC in March 1865, he musters out of the army at Camp Dennison. He returns home to Alexander and is a farmer and railroad section boss. He dies on July 17, 1910.]

Amos Hartdorn, Co. H. 22nd Regt VRC, No. 5 Elizabeth Street, Newark, NJ [8th New Jersey Infantry–Standing 5 feet, 6½ inches tall, he enrolls at Newark, New Jersey in September 1861. At the battle of the Wilderness in 1864, he is shot in the right knee and is treated at Finley Hospital in Washington. Unable to return to his regiment, he is transferred to the VRC in 1864. In 1865, he is court-martialed for absence without leave, and is confined for two months at hard labor. He is discharged at Camp Chase, Ohio in 1865. After the war, he lives in Newark and Riverdale, New Jersey, and is employed as a silver plater. He marries Hilda Conrad in 1871 and has three children— Laura Hilda, August A. and Walter H. Hartdorn. He dies in Jacksonville Beach, Florida, on Jan. 27, 1932, at the age of 91.]

Charles B. Hinchman, No. 1027
Callowhill Street, Philadelphia, Penna.

Fromton Allen, Croton,
Lee County, Iowa

Leonard Grose, Old Town Maine *[16th*
Maine Infantry—Stands 5 feet, 5½ inches
tall. At Spottsylvania, Virginia, in 1864, he
is shot in the head, five inches from his right
eye, fracturing the skull. He is paralyzed for
two weeks, and while eventually recovering,
sports a droopy left eyelid. He is treated at
Fredericksburg for a few days and then is sent
to Mount Pleasant U.S. General Hospital in
Washington. In 1864, during the Confeder-
ate raid on Washington, he catches a cold
which leads to pain, "particularly before a
storm, extending down the arm & along the
collar bone," he writes. He transfers to the
22nd VRC. After his discharge, he returns
to Oldtown, Maine, where he earns a living
as a logger and house carpenter. He marries
Sarah Ryder, but divorces in 1888. His second
wife is Frances Isabelle Pinkham, and they
have three children: Leonard Ray, Benita
Frances and Howard Cecil Grose. Leonard
dies at age 74 on Nov. 4, 1911, at South Gardiner, Maine.]

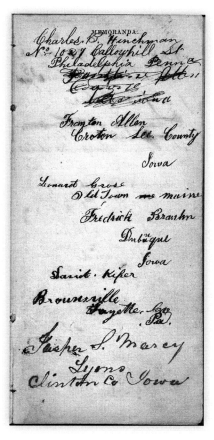

Frederick Brauhn, Dubuque, Iowa. *[21st Iowa Infantry—*
Suffering from chronic diarrhea during the Siege of Vicksburg,
he is treated in 1863 at the Gayoso General Hospital in Memphis,
Tennessee. Later he is sent to Benton Barracks in St. Louis with
fever and inflamed lungs, and thence to Lawson General Hospital
and Jefferson Barracks near St. Louis. He transfers to the VRC
in June 1864, and in the winter of 1865 he and Ephraim help
guard substitutes en route to City Point, Virginia. They are ar-
rested by military authorities in Baltimore on Jan. 8, 1865 on
charges of defrauding their escorts, and are confined for more
than two months until they are released. He marries Magdalena
P. Hess in 1872, and their three children are Mary Louisa, Anna

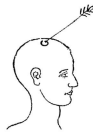

Surgeon's sketch of the
skull wound suffered
by Leonard Grose.
[National Archives]

S. and Ida H. Braun. Plagued with pneumonia, he dies in Dubuque on Feb. 22, 1883.]

David Kifer, Brownsville, Fayette Co., Pa. [62nd Pennsylvania Infantry—Standing 5 feet, 7½ inches tall, he joins the army as a substitute for Daniel Delaney of Brownsville, Pennsylvania. He suffers from bunions on the soles of his feet and spends most of the war sick in Washington military hospitals. He transfers to the VRC in August 1864 and is discharged at Camp Dennison in August 1865. After the war, he resides in Fayette City, Bridgeport, Charleroi and California, Pennsylvania, and marries Phoebe, producing two daughters, Loetta and Margaret Kifer. They separate, but do not divorce officially until after David marries Mary Brookbank in 1874. David and Mary have eight children: Peter, Annie L., John W., James O., David E., Benjamin Harrison, Sherman Custer and Viola May Kifer. In 1885, while hauling picks in the Albany Coal Mine in Fayette County, he breaks several ribs when struck by an iron mine rail. He dies in Charleroi on Jan. 10, 1906.]

Jasper S. Marcy, Lyons, Chester co., Iowa

PART VII

Returning to Normal Life

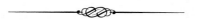

Returning to his family and friends in Kingwood,
Ephraim had to have been filled with mixed emotions, since the greatest experience of his life was now
over and quickly receding into irrelevance, as his country
wanted to get on with the business of healing and rebuilding. He rued the friendships with soldiers with
whom he had shared a suffering and had lived day to day
for months, but whom he would never see again. He had
to adjust to a new type of life as a farm laborer whose
prospect for earning a living was obstructed by deafness,
painful feet and sore back. He also faced the prospect of
answering many questions from admiring family and
friends even as he prepared to marry.

In the ensuing decades after Ephraim's return home,
the nation's collective remembrance of the war gradually
faded. Attrition took a toll as the ranks of veterans began
to die, cutting off direct sources of first hand knowledge
to be passed on to children and grandchildren. As the
Southwestern Pennsylvania region shifted toward a more
industrialized economy from its traditional agricultural
base, and eager to put the harsh wartime memories behind
them, the population's interest in the Civil War was rel-
egated to an increasing level of insignificance.

Families in the region faced more pressing issues in
the 1870s and '80s in putting clothes on their backs and
food on their tables. Among them were the expansion of
railroads, coal mining and steel production, and the related
migration into larger towns such as Connellsville, Union-

town and Pittsburgh, which provided employment paying good wages. Families were introduced to new inventions such as the telephone and light bulb, construction of engineering marvels such as tall buildings and river bridges, and concerns about stable jobs and wages in the wake of low-wage immigrant laborers, work-related injuries and deaths, brutal production schedules and the rise of organized labor unions. In the national scope, families dealt with the lure of westward expansion, the United States' centennial anniversary in 1876, another presidential assassination in 1881, racial integration, human tragedies of mass proportions such as the Haymarket Riot in Chicago and the Johnstown Flood in Pennsylvania, and the boom and bust of the economy as banks and Wall Street became more influential in manipulating the flow of capital.

Love and Marriage

On October 28, 1866, some 15 months after leaving the army, Ephraim wed his 20-year-old cousin Joanna Younkin. She was the daughter of Rev. Harmon and Susan (Faidley) Younkin and the granddaughter of John J. and Polly (Hartzell) Younkin.

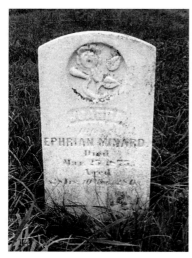

Grave of Ephraim's first wife, Joanna, in the Younkin Cemetery in Paddytown, near Kingwood. [Odger "Wayne" Miner.]

The Miners went on to have two sons—William "Lincoln" Miner and Freeman "Grant" Miner. Both were born with mental disabilities, perhaps victims of the mingling of DNA through three straight generations of inter-marriages between the Minerds and Younkins.

Sadly, their marriage only lasted for nine years. Joanna, suffering from lung fever, died on March 26, 1875, at just 28 years of age. In an obituary, the *Somerset Herald* mistakenly referred to her as "Mrs. Ephraim Weimer" but said: "We sympathize with Mr. Weimer in the loss of his partner in life, who was a member of the M.E. Church. The deceased was a lady possessing many amiable qualities." She was laid to rest in the Younkin Cemetery in nearby Paddytown. Her mis-

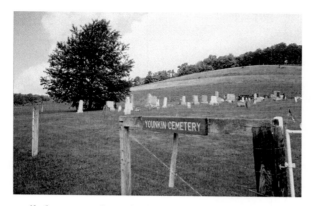

spelled grave marker, which still stands today but is badly faded, reads: "Joanna, wife of Ephrian Minard."

As a widower at age 39, and perhaps finding farming more than his feet and back could bear, Ephraim searched for a different type of work. Perhaps encouraged by his father-in-law, who was the treasurer of the Upper Turkey-foot Schools and later a salaried Turkeyfoot postmaster, Ephraim decided to pursue employment with the United States Postal Service. In March 1876, he submitted bids to carry mail three times a week from Shaff's Bridge to King-wood, a distance of 8¾ miles and back. Among his rivals for the post were his cousins Garrison N. Smith and Free-man Younkin. He was the runner-up bidder at $175, but Younkin won the work with a slightly lower bid of $173.

After spending two years alone, Ephraim married again, this time to his second cousin Rosetta Harbaugh on March 27, 1877. She was the daughter of David and Mary (Whipkey) Harbaugh of Scullton, Somerset County, and the granddaughter of Leonard and Martha (Minerd) Harbaugh Sr.

Ephraim's in-laws, Civil War veteran David Harbaugh and his wife Mary Magdalene (Whipkey).

Rosetta was some 21 years older than her husband. Ephraim Schrock and Daniel Dumbauld were witnesses to the ceremony, performed by the family's long-time friend and spiritual leader, Elder John Hickernell, founding pastor of the Old Bethel church.

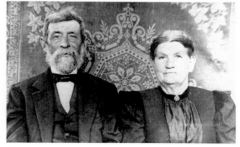

Ephraim and Rosetta with their three youngest children: John (standing), Harry and Minnie, circa 1894.

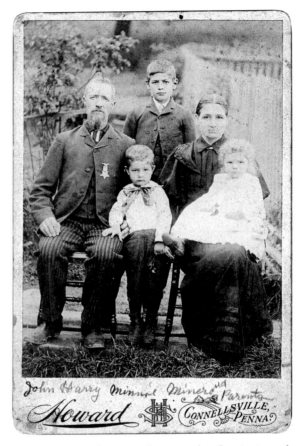

John Harry Minnie Minerald Parents
Howard   CONNELLSVILLE, PENNA

Ephraim and Rosetta knew each other intimately through their intermingled family connections over the years, as their fathers were first cousins. Ephraim and his new father in law no doubt swapped stories about their Civil War service, as David served with the 5th Pennsylvania Heavy Artillery and helped bury thousands of rotting corpses at Bull Run/Manassas.

The Miners produced three more children—John Andrew, Harry David and Minnie Edna Miner. In the early years of marriage, they resided in a log cabin near the covered bridge near Metzler's Mill. The site is along what is now Wipkey (Whipkey) Dam Road spanning Laurel Hill Creek between Scullton and Kingwood. Their eldest son John was born in the cabin.

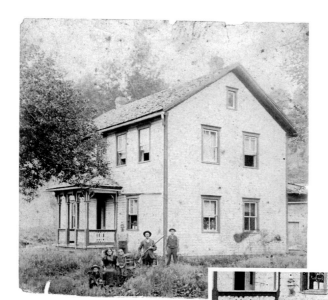

Ephraim and Rosetta (seated) in front of their new frame home in Hexebarger, circa 1896. Sons John and Harry, and daughter Minnie are also in view. The blurred figure behind young Minnie is likely either Lincoln or Grant Miner.

They later moved back to Hexebarger, where their youngest two children were born, and where they constructed a new two-story frame house in about 1896. Upon its completion, the family posed for a photograph in front of the structure. A grandson recalled proudly that Ephraim sawed all of the poplar for the house, and that there were no knots anywhere in the wood.

Now settled for good, Ephraim and Rosetta and their children led quiet, relatively insulated lives in the Somerset County mountains. Their hilly farm produced the meat and vegetables necessary for daily sustenance. Their church provided a spiritual and social outlet that kept them in regular contact with their friends. And their cousins of the Minerd, Younkin, Harbaugh and Whipkey clans were a built-in support system, devoted to helping each other in good times and bad. Granted a military pension in 1879 for his wartime injuries, Ephraim received monthly payments from the federal government for the rest of his life, providing much needed extra income.

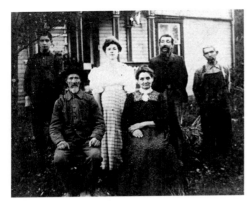

Ephraim and Rosetta, with children, l-r: Harry, Minnie, Lincoln and Grant.

A granddaughter recalled that Ephraim "spoke a lot of Dutch" [German], not bits and pieces but whole sentences and conversations," especially when he did not want nearby children to understand his words. In an era when most men were rough and tough, he was known to be quiet and gentle. Very religious, he did not allow work to be done on the farm on Sundays, and said grace before every meal, reciting the words, "From everlasting unto everlasting..."

Ephraim bore the heartache of worrying about his elder sons' ability to cope with their mental disabilities and to support themselves. The boys' grandfather, Herman Younkin, who died in the 1880s, left substantial funds for their care. In his will, he wrote: "Further I will to my grand-children namely Lincoln Minard and Grant Minard each the sum of three hundred dollars to be paid to them or their Guardians as the case may be as soon as the affairs of my estate is settled up." In 1906, Herman's widow Susan bequeathed additional funds to Linc and Grant in the amount of $25 each.

Linc had a bit of wanderlust and in 1913 made a three-week trip to Kansas and Colorado, where he claimed to have walked to the top of Pike's Peak (14,147 feet above sea level) and back again. Reported Somerset County's *Meyersdale Republican* newspaper: "Lincoln, remembering the fate of Dr. Cook, who claimed to have reached the North Pole but could not prove it, saw to it that his name was registered in the Pike's Peak News and brought a copy back to show that 'he was thar.' He was so impressed with the mountains that he now climbs one of the stupendous mountains surrounding Markleton every morning."

Ephraim's son Grant.

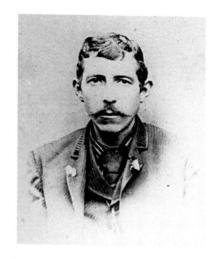

MARKLETON.

A Returned Mountain Climber.

Lincoln Miner of near here returned Wednesday from a three weeks' trip to Kansas and Colorado. He walked to the summit of Pike's Peak and returned the same way. The peak is 14,147 feet above sea level and affords a fine view. He started the ascent with a companion at 2:25 p. m., Saturday, and reached the summit between 11 and 12 o'clock at night and saw the sun rise and also a storm raging at a lower altitude. They left at 6 in the morning and reached the foot hills at 10 the same forenoon. This makes Mr Miner's third trip to Colo., and this time he was determined to reach Pike's Peak or bust." A small daily newspaper, called the Pike's Peak News, is published near the summit, in which the names of tourists climbing the mountain are registered. Lincoln, remembering the fate of Dr. Cook, who claimed to have

Grant, with more serious mental disabilities, was at times compassionate, while occasionally displaying a violent temper which frightened his nieces. In 1890, at the age of 21, Grant was so incapable of managing his own affairs that Ephraim petitioned the Court of Common Pleas to be named his guardian and to receive an allowance to cover "boarding, clothing, care and attention until further order of the court." Later, the Somerset Trust Company was named guardian of Grant's finances.

The final 25 years of Ephraim's life were filled with all of the activities of a normal family—marriages, funerals, births of grandchildren, faithful church attend-

Left: *Meyersdale Republican* article about Linc's walk to the top of Pike's Peak, 1913. [Meyersdale Public Library]

Above: Ephraim's son Lincoln.

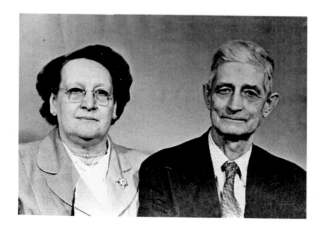

Ephraim's son Harry and his wife Amanda.

Ephraim's son John and his wife Susie.

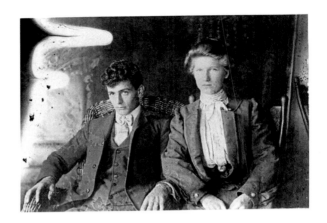

Ephraim's daughter Minnie and her husband Jacob Gary.

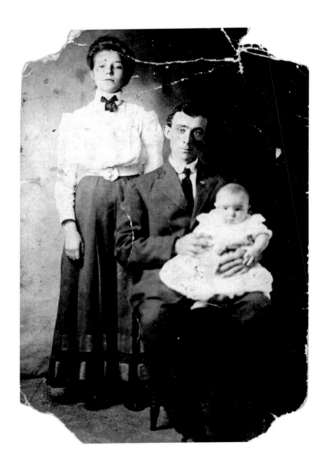

ance, barn building, and visits with family and friends. Son John married Susie Pletcher and had seven children, son Harry wed Amanda "Mandy" Burkett and produced a daughter and son, and daughter Minnie married Jacob A. "Jake" Gary and had 12 children.

To generate income, Ephraim and Rosetta sold their farm produce door to door in nearby towns. They had regular customers who put in weekly orders for vegetables and milk. Grandchildren helped prepare the foodstuffs for market, including wrapping individual onions in paper to be sold for a few cents apiece. In a good week they generated $30 for their efforts.

While usually mild-mannered, Ephraim occasionally flashed his temper. Grandson Victor Clyde Miner recalled an incident when the two were working together in a flour mill Ephraim had built. Victor, perhaps not even age five, accidentally mixed some chaff into a pile of otherwise finely-ground flour. Upon discovering the mistake, Ephraim became angry, and called his grandson a "dirty rascal." The boy later asked his mother what a "rascal" was, and when told it meant someone who stirred up trouble, the boy's feelings were hurt to think that his grandfather had used such strong language on him.

Another time, when grandchildren complained of hunger, he retorted: "You don't know what it means to be hungry. When I was in the Civil War we were so hungry that if I had seen a piece of meat lying in the mud I would have eaten it."

Ephraim and Rosetta mourned when son John and wife Susie lost two infants—Ethel (1903) and Harold (1911)—whose tender remains rest in the Old Bethel Church of God cemetery. They also grieved for son Linc, who was briefly married to Alice Pearl Ohler but came home one day to an empty house. His wife had packed up their young son Melvin and household goods and moved away.

PART VIII

Civil War Reunions and Final Years

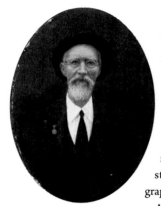

Above: Ephraim in later years.

The GAR medal.

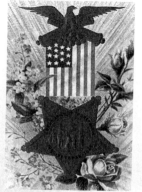

In the 1880s, having relished two decades of peace, the nation underwent a resurgence of Civil War interest. A veterans' organization, known as the Grand Army of the Republic, was formed nationally to lobby for greater pension benefits and to promote like-minded candidates for political office. By 1890, the GAR's membership roster had swelled to 400,000 nationally, with Ephraim becoming a member in good stead. He proudly sported his GAR medal in photographs over the years.

As well, monuments began to be erected on Civil War battle sites in the 1880s, and histories of individual regiments were published in growing numbers. President Harrison signed a law in 1890 establishing the first national military park at Chickamauga, in response to a heavy lobbying effort by veterans of that battle. Other national military parks were authorized during the 1890s at Gettysburg, Shiloh and Vicksburg.

That groundswell of enthusiasm may have truly validated Ephraim's wartime experience for the first time, both in the pension compensation he received, and in the public's appreciation for the service that he and his colleagues had rendered, without regard to the specifics of his particular story. It was no longer important that he and the 142nd Pennsylvania had been routed at Fredericksburg, or that he had spent two-and-a-half years in Army hospitals and in light duty assignments. What was significant in the eyes of the community was that he had been there at all, that he put his life on the line, and had suffered enduring injuries, and that he was still alive and available to be widely appreciated in person.

In 1889, a monument to the 142nd Pennsylvania was dedicated at Gettysburg. Ephraim is believed to have traveled there with fellow veterans for the unveiling of the distinctive cross-shaped memorial. While he may inwardly have cringed with regret at having missed the battle, it would not have mattered as much to his fellow veterans, and the public at large would never have known.

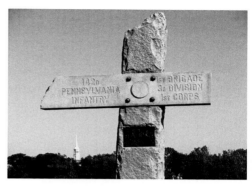

Top: Monument to the 142nd Pennsylvania at Gettysburg, on Reynolds Avenue, dedicated with pomp and circumstance in 1889. [Author photo.]

A year later, in 1890, a history of his regiment was published in the book *War History*, authored by former commanding officer Horatio Warren, reprinting many of the speeches made at the Gettysburg dedication. Ephraim's name was printed in the slim burnt-orange covered volume, in a roster of soldiers, as were the names of Martin Miner and Andrew Jackson Rose and other friends. Ephraim purchased a copy, and treasured it for the rest of his life. Seeing his name in print in a book was further sanctification of his experience and sacrifices.

History of the 142nd Pennsylvania, *War History*, authored by Col. Horatio N. Warren. Ephraim bought a copy which was passed down to his son Harry.

He relished attending annual regimental reunions throughout the region. In the process, he became a minor celebrity as his name often was published by local newspapers in lists of the attendees. At an 1918 event, the *Somerset Herald* named him among "a remarkable assemblage of aged men" who had gathered in the courthouse in Somerset, and at the "conclusion of the speeches the 121 aged veterans fell in line, and preceded by the Sons of Veterans' Drum Corps, marched to the Christian church, where a banquet was served..."

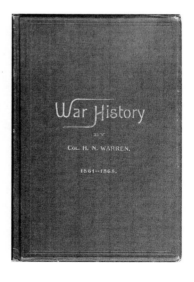

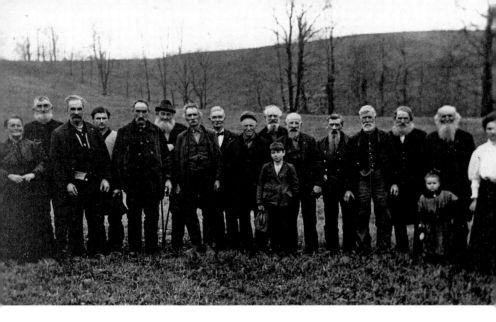

Ephraim's cousin Martin Miner, 9th from left, and fellow Civil War veterans of Normalville, Pennsylvania. Martin's step brother Michael A. Firestone, a wounded member of the 142nd Pennsylvania, also may be in this image.

The effect of this veneration in the minds of veterans cannot be understated, and often was framed in Christian terms which Ephraim held so dearly in his heart. At the 1893 reunion, which he and his cousins attended, their former commander Horatio Warren spoke these moving words, later republished in the Connellsville newspaper:

The outside world sometimes wonders why old soldiers love each other so dearly. It is because in three years we lived a lifetime, shoulder to shoulder. You fought to save me, I fought to save you, and we both fought to save our country. God smiled upon us and gave us the victory at last. Today as we rejoice our hearts become young again. In our imagination we go through the long marches, drenched by the rain and chilled by snow, we stand on picket mount at night and then again we see our comrades struggling in the throes of death. All around us they fall by our side, some maimed for life and others receiving the fatal shot that calls their soul to God. We wondered then and wonder now why we were saved and they were taken. After the smoke of battle had lifted we saw their bodies cold and lifeless upon the ground. We wonder why it was and remember that Jesus Christ died to make men holy and they died to make men free.

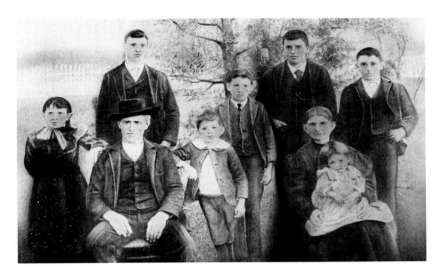

When the Pennsylvania Memorial was dedicated at Gettysburg in September 1910, Ephraim was among 37 county men to attend, with free transportation provided by the state. He again was named in newspaper articles about the event.

Ephraim remained active socially as he aged into his 60s and 70s, despite his inability to hear well. In October 1905, his beloved 65-year-old cousin Martin Miner and his wife Amanda spent an enjoyable weekend visiting with Ephraim and Rosetta and other family and friends in Kingwood. While there, Martin visited his birthplace at Hexebarger but after returning home told a *Connellsville Courier* reporter that the "old ear marks of boyhood days are about all obliterated." After a veterans' reunion in Washington, D.C., in October 1915, Ephraim received the sad news that Martin had dropped dead after returning home, having marched in the grand review before President Woodrow Wilson. Within an hour after arriving home, said a newspaper, "supper had just been finished and the veteran had pushed back his chair and was relating events of the grand encampment when he suddenly collapsed and within a few minutes was dead from apoplexy." The newspaper reported that Martin had:

> ...joined the veterans from this section when they departed in a special car on Monday. Throughout the trip he appeared in the best of spirits, and companions

Ephraim's cousin Martin Miner, seated with his wife Amanda, holding baby Nettie, and children, L-R: Agnes, Warren, Ed, Charles, George and John, of Normalville, Pennsylvania.

MARCHES IN GRAND REVIEW; RETURNS HOME; DROPS DEAD

Martin Miner, Normalville
Veteran, Victim of
Apoplexy.

SERVED IN THE 142ND INFANTRY

Accompanied Civil War Soldiers Who
Went from Here to the G. A. R. Re-
union at Washington and was in
Best of Spirits During the Trip.

Mart——e Miner, a Civil War veteran
of Normalville, attended the Grand
Army of the Republic reunion in
Washington, marched in the grand review before President Wilson, returned home and dropped dead after eat-
ing supper last night. He was a
victim of apoplexy.
    Mr. Miner was 75 years old. He
joined the veterans from this section
when they departed in a special car on
Monday. Throughout the trip he appeared in the best of spirits, and com-
panions say he apparently showed no
ill effects of the long hike up Pennsylvania avenue. On the return trip the
party was delayed several hours be-

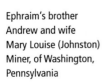

Connellsville Daily Courier coverage of the unexpected death of Ephraim's cousin Martin. [Carnegie Free Library of Connellsville]

say he apparently showed no ill effects of the long hike up Pennsylvania avenue. On the return trip the party was delayed several hours because of a freight wreck near Williams, and he was a day late arriving home. It is believed reaction from the excitement of the reunion and the journey home resulted fatally.

Ephraim's aged brother Andrew and wife Mary Louse once traveled for a visit from their home in Washington, Pennsylvania, as described in the introduction to this book. They enjoyed each other's company so much that it made an impression on Ephraim's daughter, and she recounted it more than 60 years later in her one and only conversation with the author. The photograph of the two couples together later helped plant the seeds for creation of the Minerd.com website, our national reunion and this volume.

Ephraim was an active traveler, visiting his cousin Sadie (Minerd) Luckey in Dawson and his sister Nancy Farabee in Waynesburg. One of Nancy's grandsons, Donnus Franklin Farabee, recalled a visit Ephraim made to the Farabee home in Waynesburg, circa 1911, when Ephraim was age 73, and Nancy 63. The grandson, then a boy, sat with the aged uncle, and listened

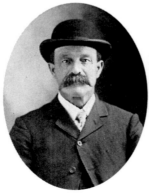
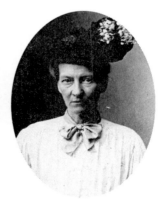

Ephraim's brother Andrew and wife Mary Louise (Johnston) Miner, of Washington, Pennsylvania

to everything he said. Upon preparing to leave, Ephraim turned down Nancy's offer for coffee despite the cold day, preferring instead a cup of hot water. Together, Ephraim, his sister Nancy and their brother Andrew attended the 1913 Minerd Reunion at Ohiopyle, Pennsylvania, along with more than 120 of their cousins from throughout the region.

Ephraim's beloved sister, Nancy Farabee, on the porch of her home in Waynesburg, Pennsylvania.

In August 1920, just seven months before his death, Ephraim took his young grandson Norman Gary to the clan's reunion at the Ferncliff Hotel in Ohiopyle. In reporting on the gathering, the *Connellsville Daily Courier* said Ephraim "is a veteran of the Civil War and is the oldest representative of the Minerd family."

In 1917, at the outbreak of World War I, the 79-year-old Ephraim remarked wistfully that he wished he could enlist and serve his country again.

Artifacts from the 1920 Minerd-Miner reunion at Ferncliff Hotel at Ohiopyle, Pennsylvania, including an article in the *Connellsville Daily Courier*.

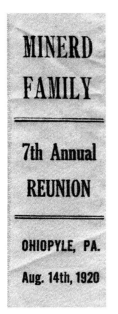

MINERD FAMILY

7th Annual

REUNION

OHIOPYLE, PA.

Aug. 14th, 1920

Minerd Reunion.

Ohiopyle was the scene of a large and happy gathering Saturday when members of the Minerd family assembled for their eighth annual reunion. Rev. D. E. Minerd of Dunbar delivered the principal address of the day. At noon an elaborate dinner was served. The next reunion will be held on the second Saturday in August, 1921 at Ohiopyle. Among the guests present were Mr. and Mrs. Ephriam Minerd of Markleton. The former is a veteran of the civil War and is the oldest representative of the Minerd family. Mr. and Mrs. C. S. Freed and daughter, Miss Mary of Dunbar township; Mr. and Mrs. J. D. Minerd and Mr. and Mrs. Silas Minerd of Connellsville, were also guests.

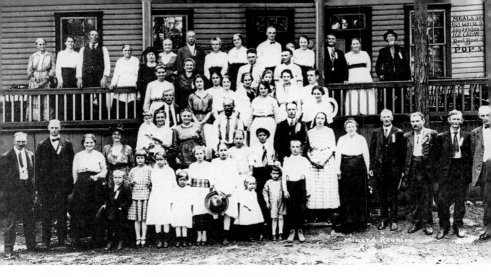

1920 Minerd-Miner reunion at Ohiopyle. In the photo, Ephraim stands at far right on the porch, with his young grandson Norman Gary in the first row, 4th from left.

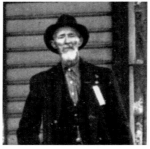

Ephraim passed away at home on March 11, 1921, at the age of 83. Members of his Civil War Post were unable to attend the funeral at the family dwelling due to the "almost impassible condition of the roads," said a Somerset newspaper. At his insistence, there were no flowers but rather flags at his funeral, and as requested he was buried at the Kingwood IOOF Cemetery, in his Army uniform, with its buttons polished brightly.

EPHRAIM MINER.

Ephraim Miner, a veteran of the Civil War, and a citizen of Upper Turkeyfoot township, died at his home Friday morning, March 11th, at 5 o'clock at the age of 83 years, 6 months, and 10 days. Mr. Miner was a son of the late Henry Miner of Upper Turkeyfoot township, and a life long citizen of this township. He has been ailing and in failing health for several years, and his death is due to old age and a complication of diseases.

The subject of these remarks was a private in Company D, 142nd Regiment Pennsylvania Volunteers, and for many years a member of the G. A. R. Post No. 210 of Somerset. He was enrolled into the country's service on the 1st day of August, 1862, and discharged from the service on the 1st day of July, 1865, being a pensioner for many years, and during the last six months made application for total disability pension of $72 per month.

Mr. Miner was twice married. On the 28th day of October, 1866, he was married to Joanna Younkin, daughter of the late Herman Younkin of Upper Turkeyfoot township, she departing this life on the 25th

Ephraim's lengthy obituary in the *Somerset County Leader.*

Right: Final resting place for Ephraim and Rosetta at the Odd Fellows Cemetery in Kingwood.

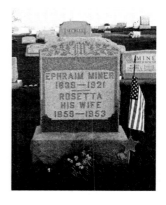

Rosetta's Years as a Widow

Rosetta outlived her husband by more than three decades, remaining in their home in Hexebarger, and surrounded by a growing brood of grandchildren and great-grandchildren. In August 1924, she and sons John and Harry and their families were among 82 relatives and friends who attended the Minerd-Miner reunion in Confluence. Of that event, the *Meyersdale Republican* reported: "A very successful and pleasant reunion of the Minard family was held in what is known locally as Lincoln's grove, near the Western Maryland Railroad Station.... The family is a numerous one in Western Pennsylvania...."

Rosetta enjoyed attending reunions of her own Harbaugh family. She and her children and grandchildren went to the first event in 1926, honoring her mother Mary's 94th birthday, at her sister Susie Conn's house on the old Harbaugh homestead. The several hundred attendees posed for a wide panorama photograph.

A photo of the 1929 Harbaugh Reunion at the Jersey Church near Ursina shows her standing with her mother and sisters Susie Conn, Sadie Ream, Letitia Stoner and Lucinda Younkin Johnson. At the 1936 event, she posed with more than 110 cousins at the Kingwood Odd Fellows Grove. She received the "Oldest Woman Present" award various years from 1947 to 1951. The Harbaugh Reunions continue today in Farmington, Pennsylvania, with their archives published on Minerd.com.

Rosetta's nephew, Charles Arthur Younkin (nicknamed "Charleroi Charley"), was a genealogy researcher, writer and

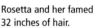

Rosetta and her famed 32 inches of hair.

Large gathering in 1926 for the 94th birthday of Rosetta's mother, Mary Magadalene (Whipkey) Harbaugh, at the old Harbaugh homestead near Clairton Lake, Somerset County. Rosetta sits at left of center, between her mother and sister Susie Conn.

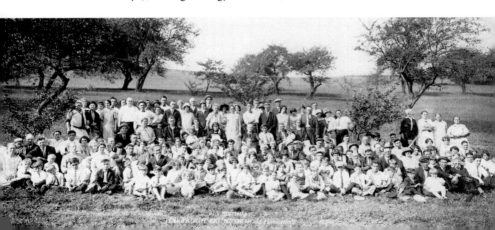

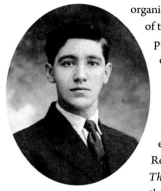

Charles A. Younkin, of Charleroi, Pennsylvania, whose interview with his aunt Rosetta in 1935 furnished valuable insights into Ephraim's boyhood experiences.

organizer of the Younkin National Home-Coming Reunions of the 1930s and early '40s. He published a related newspaper, the *Younkin Family News Bulletin,* which had a distribution to Younkins coast to coast.

On September 2, 1934, when the Younkin clan held its initial reunion at the Kingwood Picnic Grove, and drew 400 guests, Ephraim's son Grant was first on the scene. Writing in a manuscript history of the event, Grant's cousin and reunion president Otto Roosevelt Younkin said:

The sky was clear, the air slightly cool, a fine day for the reunion. The first to arrive was Grant Miner, of Ursina Pa, who was upon the ground by 8 o'clock. By noon quite a number had assembled and partook of a bounteous basket-dinner.

In October 1935, he traveled for an overnight visit with his aunt Rosetta to interview her about the tangled connections between the Minerd, Harbaugh and Younkin families. Her stories clarified many confusing relationships and lit the fires of his imagination. He later summarized them in a letter to a cousin, perhaps the only documentation of ancient and silent genealogical connections.

In the 1940s, Rosetta resided with her son Harry in Connellsville. At the age of 83, in 1942, Rosetta traveled to Oblong, Illinois to visit her ailing sister, Letitia (Harbaugh) Stoner, who had suffered a massive stroke and was left paralyzed. She returned home safely, as Harry gratefully penned in his diary.

On Sept. 23, 1953, at the age of 94, Rosetta passed away at the home of her son John and his wife Susie along the Springfield Pike in neighboring Fayette County. Her remains were brought to Kingwood to be placed at rest beside her husband, after a separation of more than three decades.

Her double-cousin Albert "Ward" Minerd, of Mill Run, Fayette County, noted her funeral in his diary on Sept. 26, 1953, writing: "Rossette Harbaugh Miner was burried today."

Over the ensuing decades, Ephraim and Rosetta's grandchildren and great-grandchildren swelled in number and scattered all across the United States. A handful of offspring held a reunion in 1986 at the Kingwood Odd Fellows Grove in Kingwood. That first reunion evolved into what is now the national Minerd-Minard-Miner-Minor Reunion. After two decades at the Kingwood grove, the reunion was moved to the Indian Creek Valley Community Center near Indian Head, Fayette County.

Ephraim's newspaper obituaries have been reprinted over the years in local historical publications. The *Somerset County Leader* piece was published in the book, *Down the Road of Our Past* in the 1990s, produced by the Rockwood Historical Society. The *Somerset Herald* obit appears in the November 2005 edition of the *Laurel Messenger* newsletter of the Historical and Genealogical Society of Somerset County. As well, Ephraim and Rosetta are named in the 2010 historical novel *A Place Called Hexie,* authored by Samuel G. Miller.

On July 26, 2003, a granite and bronze monument to the 142nd Pennsylvania was unveiled beside the Somerset County Courthouse, presented by the 142nd Pennsylvania Volunteer Infantry Living Historians and through the generosity of the community. The primary address was made by John Heiser, ranger and historian at the Gettysburg National

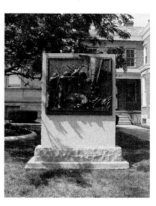

Monument to the 142nd Pennsylvania Infantry standing today at the Somerset County Courthouse.

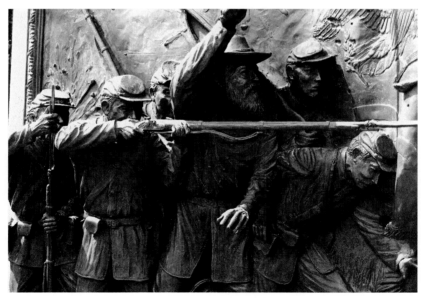

Military Park. Sculpted by Wayne Hyde of Mann's Choice, Pennsylvania, the monument depicts the regiment's counter-attack at Gettysburg and the look of determination on the soldiers' faces.

The Slaughter Pen Farm in Fredericksburg, where Ephraim fought, and upon which his friends were wounded and died, was in private ownership for many years, and at one point it was on the selling block to be converted into an industrial site.

A consortium of funders, led by the Civil War Preservation Trust, raised millions of dollars to purchase the land in 2006. Joining the effort were the National Park Service, Commonwealth of Virginia, Central Virginia Battlefields Trust and SunTrust Banks, Inc. Their mission: "to save this land forever as a gift to the nation."

Conclusion

In a dramatic era of social, political and economic upheaval driven by vast bloodshed, Ephraim Miner came into manhood during the Civil War with his own horror, heartache and physical sacrifice. By all accounts, the course of his life was forever altered by his experience away in military service, and he never lived a day afterward without feeling its physical affect. The conflict refined his values and character as a husband, father and grandfather, as a productive farmer and as an exemplary citizen of his community even as he endured other significant emotional and physical suffering throughout the rest of his years.

Given Americans' relatively short attention span, it is remarkable that Ephraim is remembered at all in the 21st century. Today his offspring are in the sixth generation of descendants. His grandchildren whom I interviewed over the years, unfortunately now dead, had stories to tell. Even today some of his great-grandchildren hold his name in esteem, despite all of the assaults that time and distractions ravage on memory. Yet his wartime story largely has been forgotten, mirroring the tendency of following generations to focus on the concerns of the here and now while allowing the details of the past to fade away.

The Minerd.com website and *Well At This Time* volume are designed to fulfill the charge made by my Aunt Jessie (Miner) Schultz to "find out about" Ephraim and his people. These devices of mass communication bring his story back to life in ways that can be easily enjoyed and preserved for future generations of family, friends and Civil War enthusiasts. This book certainly has made me a much deeper admirer of the man I first saw in an old photograph, many years ago.

Ephraim's story is instructive for today's generation. He stood up and took a stand for an unpopular cause which had divided our nation but in which he believed. He paid a stiff price. And in the end, he and his nation were—and all of us are—the better for his steely resolve.

END NOTES

Introduction

13. "In 1989, at my request, Pennsylvania Congressman Doug Walgren wrote to ..." Walgren, Douglas. Letter to Wynema E. Smith, Chief ABCMR, Department of the Army Reserve Personnel Center, St. Louis, Mo. Jan. 17, 1989.

13-14. "So in May 2000, I launched the Minerd.com website..." Mark A. Miner, Minerd. com Web Site.

14. "As I wrote in *Pittsburgh Quarterly Magazine* in 2008, on the 250th anniversary of the founding of Pittsburgh..." Mark A. Miner, "Family Is Everything," *Pittsburgh Quarterly Magazine*, Fall 2008.

Part I - Becoming a Man

20. "He was an eyewitness to a triple tragedy involving his mother Polly..." Charles Arthur Younkin, letter to Otto Roosevelt Younkin, October 15, 1935.

20. "One day grandfather and grandson went hunting together for game..." Ibid.

21. "A second tragedy, a fire that destroyed the Minerd home, crippled Ephraim's father economically..." Edward John Miner, conversation with the author, October 29, 1978.

21. "By 1860, the year before the war erupted, Ephraim's parents and siblings moved to the northern panhandle of Virginia..." 1860 Census of the United States, Upper Turkeyfoot Township, Somerset County, Pa., Roll M653_1183; Page 645; Image:653; Family History Library Film 805183. Also see 1860 U.S. Census of Marshall County, Va., Roll M653_1360, Page 325, Image 333; Family History Library Film 805360.

21. "At the age of 20 or 21, moved by the preaching and worship at the newly built Old Bethel..." *Somerset Herald*, March 1921.

21. "Old Bethel, with its roots in the German Reformed Church, ..." C.H. Forney, *History of the Churches of God in the United States of North America*. Harrisburg, Pennsylvania: The Publishing House of the Churches of God, 1914.

21. "He stood 5 feet, 10 inches tall, had dark eyes and dark hair, and a fair complexion..." Ephraim Miner, United States Military Record, National Archives Building, Washington, D.C.

22-23. "After this call I was uneasy, I felt I ought to enlist, why I did not immediately it is..." Edwin R. Gearhart, *Reminiscences of the Civil War*. Stroudsburg, Pa., Daily Record Press, 1901, p. 7.

23. "Two weeks after the draft law was passed, when he was age 24,..." Ephraim Miner, United States Military Record, National Archives Building, Washington, D.C.

23. "After arriving, they marched to the state capitol building, where their eyes beheld the great dome..." Gearhart, p. 17.

23. "[They] represented the diverse pursuits and composite character of the American citizen..." Warren, Horatio Nelson, *Two Reunions of the 142d Regiment, Pa. Vols.*, also known as *War History*, Buffalo, N.Y., The Courier Company, 1890, p. 49.

24. "We learned from the wounded, who were flocking into the city..." Ibid, p. 14.

24. "'This was our first picket duty,' Warren writes..." Ibid., p. 15.

24-25. "For the first time, these raw men observed 'the horrible results of these battles'..." Ibid., p. 16.

25. "Reports Warren, 'This march was fraught with much that was trying to our experience'..." Ibid., p. 17.

25. "Ephraim and his mates stood in snow one inch deep, and as each one..." Gearhart, p. 23.

25. "As Meade rode by, they made loud catcalls at him for 'crackers and hard-tack'..." Warren, p. 17.

26. "Gearhart writes that while in the camp, the men cooked for themselves using a standard-issue..." Gearhart, p. 24.

Part II - First Action at Fredericksburg

27. "Tony Horwitz's *Confederates in the Attic*..." Tony Horwitz, *Confederates in the Attic*, New York: Vintage Books, a Division of Random House, Inc., 1998, p. 229.

27. "Shelby Foote, in *The Civil War: A Narrative*, writes that..." Shelby Foote, *The Civil War: A Narrative, Fredericksburg to Meridian*. New York: Random House, 1963, p. 20.

28. "[It was where] our first genuine experience of war commenced..." Warren, p. 18.

29. "*In This Hallowed Ground*, author Bruce Catton writes '... the hills are just high enough'...," Bruce Catton, *This Hallowed Ground*, Garden City, N.Y.: Doubleday & Company, Inc., 1956, p. 188.

29. "On the morning of December 10, Ephraim and his mates in camp near town were awakened...," Gearhart, p. 24.

29. "Here we had an unobstructed view of the flat lying between us and the river...," Ibid.

31. "The enemy's position was so strong that a Confederate artillerist...," Carl Sandburg, *Abraham Lincoln: The War Years*, Volume I, New York: Harcourt, Brace & World, Inc., 1939, p. 629.

31. "Pulitzer Prize winning author Douglas Southall Freeman calls it a 'swirling silver'...," Douglas Southall Freeman, *Lee's Lieutenants, A Study in Command*. New York: Charles Scribner's Sons, 1942-1944 p. 348.

31. "...while Catton describes '... a heavy wet fog along the river'...," Bruce Catton, *Glory Road*, Garden City, N.Y.: Doubleday & Company, Inc., 1952, p. 34.

31. "Gearhart writes of 'A thick fog covered the plain'...," Gearhart, p. 25.

31. "Writes Catton: 'So the guns opened, and a tremendous cloud'...," Bruce Catton, *Glory Road*, p. 37.

32-33. "Viewing this carnage from afar, Lee was moved to utter...," Bruce Catton, *Lee*: An Abridgement in One Volume by Richard Harwell. New York: Simon & Schuster Inc., 1997. p. 278.

33. "Burnside watched in anguish as his divisions were obliterated...," Shelby Foote, *The Civil War: Fredericksburg to Meridian,* p. 42.

33. "McCalmont, in temporary leadership of the 142nd Pennsylvania...," Gearhart, p. 25.

34. "As the 142nd Pennsylvania began to march, they saw that...," Ibid.

34. "They saw the first of the day's dreadful sights...," Gearhart, p. 26.

34. "The Pennsylvanians surged toward tracks...." Details of the 142nd Pennsylvania in action is well described in *The Federicksburg Campaign* by Francis Augustín O'Reilly (pp. 139-216), *Fredericksburg! Fredericksburg!* by George C. Rable (pp. 210-217). See also descriptions of the federal breakthrough in Foote's *The Civil War: A Narrative, Fredericksburg to Meridian* (pp. 36-37), Freeman's *Lee's Lieutenants* (pp. 353-358) and Catton's *Glory Road* (pp. 43-46).

34. "For a short time they 'made great headway, crumpling up a couple'...," Catton, *Glory Road,* p. 45.

34-35. "In *The Fredericksburg Campaign,* Francis Augustín O'Reilly notes that...," O'Reilly, p. 505.

35. "At one point the men were commanded to 'Fix bayonets, forward, charge,'...," Gearhart, p. 26.

36. "One 142nd Pennsylvania member writes of seeing 'a terrific and most galling'...," Rable, p. 210.

36. "Michael A. Firestone was shot through the hip and thigh and Jacob Pritts was hit in the shin...," Michael A. Firestone, Civil War Pension File, National Archives Building, Washington, D.C., Application #117033, Certificate #79017, Widow Application #1143973, Certificate #879930. See also Jacob Pritts, Civil War Pension File, National Archives Building, Washington, D.C., Application #163879, Certificate #114822.

36. "Among the members of Ephraim's Company C to be killed outright were David Ansell...," Warren, pp. 69-70.

36. "Writes Gearhart, "[The] balls were whizzing, shells bursting'...," Gearhart, p. 27.

37. "English historian George Francis Robert Henderson counted...," George F. R. Henderson, *The Campaign of Fredericksburg, Nov.-Dec., 1862.* London: Kegal Paul, Trench & Co., 1886, p. 82.

37. "Snowden of the 142nd Pennsylvania writes: 'The sacrifice was in vain'...," Warren, p. 51.

37. "Sandburg writes that some of the wounded 'lay forty-eight hours'...," Sandburg, p. 629.

37-38. "Says Freeman, 'The horror of the scene was far greater at close range'...," Freeman, *Lee,* p. 281.

38. "Another soldier observed that a Pennsylvania man, badly wounded in the leg...," Walt Whitman, *Complete Prose Works,* Philadelphia: David McKay, Publisher, 1892, p. 28.

38. "The night 'brought a storm of sleet and driving rain'...," Foote, T*he Civil War, Fredericksburg to Meridian,* p. 44.

38. "In his report to his superior officer, Major General Henry Halleck, Burnside defended...," *New York Herald,* Dec. 18, 1862, p. 1.

39. "Gearhart recalls seeing his regiment there:...," Gearhart, p. 30.

40. "In summarizing their emotional anguish, Gearhart recalls that when they first prepared...," Gearhart, p. 33.

40. "...hundreds of the worst wounded men I have ever seen...," Percy Harold Epler, *The Life of Clara Barton*, New York: The Macmillan Company, 1915, p. 66.

40. "Her biographer, Percy Harold Epler, states that she 'moved among them'...," Ibid., p. 68.

40. "While crossing the river to tend to wounded there, she was being assisted by...," Ibid., pp. 69-70.

41. "The results of the late battle are exhibited everywhere...," Whitman, p. 26.

41. "...the hall was full of these wrecks of humanity...," Louisa May Alcott, *Hospital Sketches*, Boston: James Redpath, Publisher, 1863, p. 28.

42. "The outcome had serious aftershocks in the nation's collective psyche...," J.G. Randall and David Herbert Donald. *The Civil War and Reconstruction*, 2nd Ed. Lexington, Massachusetts: D.C. Heath and Company, 1969, p. 225.

Part III - Leaving the Regiment for Medical Care

44. "One granddaughter recalled the significant pain he endured...," Evanell (Miner) Kimmel Nicklow, interview with the author, Kingwood, Pa., July 22, 1989.

44. "A closer parallel may be drawn from comrade Aaron Zufall...," Joseph K. Barnes, *Medical and Surgical History of the War of the Rebellion*, Part III, Vols. I and II, prepared by Charles Smart, Washington, D.C.: United States Government Printing Office, 1888, p. 654.

46. "Walt Whitman described Finley Hospital as...," Whitman, p. 47.

46. "Said one narrative, it was 'perhaps the largest and most complete Army Hospital'...." This quote is taken from the caption of a Civil War era print published by James D. Gay now in the collection of the Library Company of Philadelphia, entitled "Satterlee U.S.A. General Hospital, West Philadelphia."

47. "An anonymous Sister wrote that in addition to Catholics...," American Catholic Historical Society of Philadelphia. Records of the American Catholic Historical Society of Philadelphia, Vol. VIII, 1897, p. 402.

47. "One of them, Jerome B. Knable, wrote this entry on Aug. 1, 1863...," Diary of Corp. Jerome B. Knable, Transcript, Historical and Genealogical Society of Somerset County, Inc., n.p.

48. "Pile, a sergeant, wounded in the skull and mouth at Fredericksburg...," Simon Pile Civil War Pension File, National Archives Building, Washington, D.C., Application #189254, Certificate #128484, Widow Application #615916, Widow Certificate #418846.

49. "Never anywhere was relief and sympathy more welcome or necessary...," United States Sanitary Commission, for the Army and Navy, *First Annual Report*, Philadelphia: 1863, p. 50.

49. "At that camp, said a Christian Commission report, volunteers 'distributed wagon-loads'...," Ibid.

55. "Feb. 11-F. Iams, co D 140 P.V. ...," Frederick F. Iams Civil War Pension File, National Archives Building, Washington, D.C., Application #104267, Certificate #101962, Widow Application #848818, Widow Certificate #618371.

55. "Lincoln Hospital. He writes of 'washing and dressing wounds,' as well as providing...," Whitman, p. 45.

59. "The Canterbury music hall, on Louisiana Avenue in Washington, is a popular...," Benn Pitman, editor, *The Assassination of President Lincoln and the Trial of the Conspirators*, Cincinnati: Moore, Wilstach & Baldwin, 1865, pp. 228, 230, 345, 390.

59. "Ephraim's cousin Albert Miner, of the 19th Ohio Infantry, dies in captivity..." Mark A. Miner, Minerd.com biography of Albert Miner.

61. "Ephraim's cousin by marriage, Sylvester Georgia," Ibid., Minerd.com biography of Laveria (Minerd) Georgia.

63. "Adam Nickelson is in the 142nd Pennsylvania...," Adam Nickelson, Civil War Pension File, National Archives Building, Washington, D.C., Application #320854, Certificate #470448.

64. "In War History, Warren recalls: '[T]here emerged from the woods'...," Warren, p. 28.

64. "Writes Warren: "The woods here were afire'...," Ibid., p. 29.

64. "At the battle of Resaca, Georgia, Ephraim's cousin Daniel L. Minor...," Mark A. Miner, Minerd.com biography of Daniel L. Minor.

65. "Walt Whitman visits the capitol building occasionally, saying...," Whitman, p. 63.

65. "Writes Warren: 'We had closed up our ranks and were marching in fours'...," Warren, p. 32.

66. "Warren writes: '[B]y reason of the stubbornness of the enemy's rear-guard'...," Ibid, p. 31.

67. "In addition to protecting the nation's capitol, Slough's charge is to prevent...," *Reports of Committees of the Senate of the United States, for the Third Session of the Thirty Seventh Congress*, Washington, D.C., Government Printing Office, 1863, p. 549.

67. "In *Never Call Retreat*, Catton says: 'By now the armies were running out of space'." Ibid., p. 363. Catton, *Never Call Retreat*, Garden City, N.Y.: Doubleday & Company, Inc., 1965, p. 363.

68. "...'early the next morning we found ourselves facing the same old enemy'...," Warren, p. 33.

68. "Catton says: '… a storm of Confederate rifle fire tore the Federal columns'...," Catton, *Never Call Retreat*, p. 364.

69. "During the Petersburg siege, Ephraim's cousin by marriage, Robert Rankin...," Mark A. Miner, Minerd.com biography of Hester (Minerd) Rankin.

70. "Ephraim's cousin, Leroy Bush, dies at the home of his sister...," Ibid., Minerd.com biography of Leroy Bush.

71. "As a member of the 1st Maryland Cavalry, also known as the 1st Potomac Home...," Ibid., Minerd.com biography of Martha Emma (Minerd) Gorsuch.

71. "At the battle of Monocacy Junction, Maryland, Ephraim's cousin Eli Van Horn...," Ibid., Minerd.com biography of Eli Van Horn.

73. "In *Abraham Lincoln: The War Years*, Carl Sandburg describes this battle:...," Sandburg, Vol. III, pp. 140-141.

73. "Ephraim's cousin by marriage, William J. Burditt (husband of Jemima Minerd)...," Mark A. Miner, Minerd.com biography of Jemima (Minerd) Burditt.

74. "Ephraim never mentions seeing the president, while Walt Whitman writes...," Whitman, p. 43.

75. "The VRC is created during the war to employ "worthy" convalescing and disabled soldiers...," Catton, *A Stillness At Appomattox*, Garden City, N.Y., Doubleday & Company, Inc., 1953, p. 143.

75. "At this battle, Ephraim's cousin by marriage, John Strauch...," Mark A. Miner, Minerd.com biography of Mary Hester (McKnight) Strauch.

76. "The lines all along for about five miles were in readiness at 4 a.m....," Warren, p. 38.

77. "Ephraim's cousin, Andrew Jackson Miner of the 90th Ohio Volunteer Infantry...," Mark A. Miner, Minerd.com biography of Andrew Jackson Miner of Ohio.

78. "While guarding a train in Berryville, Virginia, Ephraim's cousin Isaac Van Horn...," Ibid., Minerd.com biography of Isaac Van Horn.

78. "Ephraim's cousin, James Minerd Jr., of the 85th Pennsylvania Infantry...," Ibid., Minerd.com biography of James Minerd Jr.

79. "At Jonesboro, Georgia, Ephraim Miner's cousin Frederick Miner Jr. is injured...," Ibid., Minerd.com biography of Frederick Miner Jr.

80. "Several of Boyts' war letters later are preserved...," Somerset County (PA) Historical and Genealogical Society, Inc., "Soldiers' Letters Tell of Military," *Laurel Messenger*, May 1989, p. 355.

82. "The arsenal employs...," George R. Howell and Jonathan Tenney, *History of the County of Albany. New York*, W.W. Munsell & Co., 1886, p. 433.

84. "At Kennesaw Mountain (Big Shanty), Georgia, Ephraim's cousin Samuel Miner...," Mark A. Miner, Minerd.com biography of Samuel Miner.

89. "After the war, Joanna Minerd marries Perry Enos, a veteran...," Mark A. Miner, Minerd.com biography of Joanna (Minerd) Enos.

91. "VRC troops guard thousands of POWs at Morton...," W.H.H. Terrell, *Indiana in the War of the Rebellion*, Indianapolis, Douglass & Conner, 1869, p. 84. See also United States Christian Commission, for the Army and Navy, for the Year 1864, *Third Annual Report,* Philadelphia, April 1865, p. 141.

91. "According to Indianapolis and the Civil War, 'So many soldiers'...," John Hampden Holliday, *Indianapolis and the Civil War*, Indianapolis, Edward J. Hecker, 1911, p. 571.

91-92. "Writes Warren: '... their losses were very heavy, ours slight'...," Warren, p. 39.

93. "It was located on North Charles Street 'on the grounds of the former'...," United States Christian Commission, Third Report of the Committee of Maryland, Baltimore: James Young, 1864, p. 141.

93. "Ephraim's future nephew by marriage, Cyrus Lindley," Mark A. Miner, Minerd.com biography of Elizabeth (Miner) Lindley.

94. "More than two years before Ephraim visits there, his cousin Leonard Rowan...," Ibid., Minerd.com biography of Leonard Rowan.

Part V - The Diary for 1865

97. "While accompanying substitute soldiers on a march, Ephraim and Frederick Braun...," Ephraim Miner and Frederick Braun, Military Service Files, National Archives.

97-98. "Ephraim's cousin Alpheus Minerd, and Minerd's brother-in-law William H. Shepard...," Mark A. Miner, Minerd.com biographies of Alpheus Minerd and Sarah (Minerd) Shepard.

99. "Ephraim's friend and pen pal David Gohn is shot in the lower jaw...," David Gohn, Civil War Pension File, National Archives Building, Washington, D.C., Application #76552, Certificate #47225.

99. "Warren writes that Dabney's Mills, … 'was anything but a picnic'...," Warren, p. 40.

99. "This vote frees 15-year-old slave Fleming Woody in Virginia...," Mark A. Miner, Minerd.com biography of Susanna (Miner) Mayle Woody.

102. "Writes Warren: 'The enemy in our front were pouring in a tremendous shower'...," War History, p. 42.

103. "Warren writes: 'The next morning our forces advanced and took the South-side'...," Ibid., p. 43.

105. "Ephraim's cousin by marriage, William J. Burditt, is shot in the thigh...," Mark A. Miner, Burditt biography.

105. "Warren writes that Lee was "so completely hemmed in and surrounded...," Warren, p. 43.

105. "In a twist of fate, Custer's younger brother, Capt. Thomas Ward Custer...," Mark A. Miner, Minerd.com biographies of Rebecca (Minerd) Behme Kearns and Thomas C. Custer.

111. "Walt Whitman, watching from Pennsylvania Avenue, writes to his mother...," Whitman, Letter to Louisa Van Velsor Whitman, May 25, 1865, courtesy of the Walt Whitman Archive (www.whitmanarchive.org).

111. "The soldiers' home, previously known as Tripler Hospital in Columbus...," Jacob Henry Studer, Columbus, Ohio: Its History, Resources, and Progress, 1873, p. 75.

112. "In Ohio in the War Whitelaw Reid states: 'Through the autumn of 1864'...," Whitelaw Reid, Ohio in the War: Her Statesmen, Generals and Soldiers, Vol. I, Cincinnati, The Robert Clarke Company, 1895, pp 194-196.

113. "In response to Lincoln's assassination, June 1, 1865 is proclaimed...," William DeLoss Love Jr., Ph.D., The Fast and Thanksgiving Days of New England, Boston: Houghton, Mifflin and Company, 1895, p. 408.

116. "Having received his final pay, Ephraim makes the rail trip...," Mark A. Miner, Minerd. com biographies of Catherine (Miner) Bedillion, Chance Minor, Elias Minor, Henry Minerd, Henry Harrison Minerd, Nancy (Minor) Farabee and Susan (Miner) Birch.

121. "Both Ephraim and Harmon are mentioned in a chapter about Harman's son...," Ruth B. Reichley, *Biographical Review Containing Life Sketches of Leading Citizens of Bedford and Somerset Counties,* 1899, p. 314.

122. "Isabell Farabee is a sister of Ephraim's brother-in-law Spencer Farabee ...," Louis Thomas Farabee, *Genealogy of the Farabees in America,* Washington, D.C., 1918, p. 291.

122. "Charles and Adaline (Harbaugh) Minerd are Ephraim's uncle and aunt...," Mark A. Miner, Minerd.com biographies of Charles Minerd, Adaline (Harbaugh) Minerd, Almira Malissa (Minerd) Overholt, Josephine (Minerd) Hall, Lawson Minerd, Lucinda J. (Minerd) Hall, Martha Emma "Matt" (Minerd) Gorsuch, Rebecca "Jennie" (Minerd) Conley Woodmancy.

Part VI - Ephriam's Friends

126. "C.W. Newcomb, Pittstown, Rensselear Co., NY...," Cyrenus W. Newcomb, Civil War Pension File, National Archives Building, Washington, D.C., Application #765852, Certificate #692403.

127. "Wesley Long, East Hamburg, Erie Co., NY...," Wesley Long, Civil War Pension File, National Archives Building, Washington, D.C., Application #786397, Certificate #583993, Widow Application #591719, Widow Certificate #405337.

128. "N. Sharp, Lynn St., Clair Co., Mich....," Nelson Oscar Sharp, Civil War Pension File, National Archives Building, Washington, D.C., Application #599618, Certificate #750560, Widow Application #1133435, Widow Certificate #874722.

128. "Chauncey Brockway Esq., Nassau, Rensselear Co., NY...," Chauncey Brockway, Civil War Pension File, National Archives Building, Washington, D.C., Application #998279, Certificate #876838.

129. "George F. Rollins, Exeter, N.H. ...," George F. Rollins Civil War Pension File, National Archives Building, Washington, D.C., Application #558048, Certificate #385738, Widow Application #420379, Widow Certificate #325364.

129. "Daniel W. Ash, Ripley Po Office, Tyler Co., West Va. ...," Daniel Ash, Civil War Pension File, National Archives Building, Washington, D.C., Application #93751, Certificate #65931, Widow Application #371658, Widow Application #249817.

130. "Sylvester DeMary, Alexander, Genesee Co., NY...," Sylvester DeMary, Civil War Pension File, National Archives Building, Washington, D.C., Application #95863, Certificate #68911, Widow Application #946297, Widow Application #710967).

130. "Amos Hartdorn, Co. H. 22nd Regt VRC, No. 5 Elizabeth Street, Newark, NJ...," Amos Hartdorn Civil War Pension File, National Archives Building, Washington, D.C., Application #211141, Certificate #142871.

131. "Leonard Grose, Old Town Maine...," Leonard Grose, Civil War Pension File, National Archives Building, Washington, D.C., Application #105504, Certificate #102464, Widow Application #1072385, Widow Certificate #818758, Minor Application #1015968, Minor Certificate #795566.

131. "Frederick Brauhn, Dubuque, Iowa...," Frederick Brauhn, Civil War Pension File, National Archives Building, Washington, D.C., Application #274082, Certificate #171266, Widow Application #302325, Widow Certificate #200392.

132. "David Kifer, Brownsville, Fayette Co., Pa. ...," David Kifer, Civil War Pension File, National Archives Building, Washington, D.C., Application #822405, Certificate #609374, Widow Application #842160, Widow Certificate #636180, XC #2678251.

Part VII - Returning to Normal Life

134. "In an obituary, the *Somerset Herald* mistakenly referred to her as 'Mrs. Ephraim Weimer'...," *Somerset Herald*, March 31, 1875, p. 3.

135. "In March 1876, he submitted bids to carry mail three times a week...," *Index to the Executive Documents of the House of Representatives for the Second Session of the Forty-Fourth Congress*, Washington, D.C.: Government Printing Office, 1877, pp. 213-214.

137. "Granted a military pension in 1879 for his wartime injuries...," Ephraim Minor, Civil War Pension File, National Archives/Veterans Administration, Application #308962, Certificate #264987, Widow Application #1172852, Widow Certificate #903476, XC 2703889 (lost).

138. "A granddaughter recalled that Ephraim 'spoke a lot of Dutch'...," Kimmell Nicklow, July 1991.

138. "Very religious, he did not allow work to be done on the farm on Sundays...," Gladys (Gary) Kreger, interview with the author, Casselman, Pa., Oct. 31, 1991.

138. "The boys' grandfather, Herman Younkin, who died in the 1880s...," Herman Younkin, Somerset County Probate File, #72 of 1885.

138. "Reported Somerset County's *Meyersdale Republican* newspaper: "Lincoln, remembering the fate...," *Meyersdale Republican*, July 17, 1913.

139. "In 1890, at the age of 21, Grant was so incapable of managing...," Ephraim Miner vs. Freeman Grant Miner, Case #19 Sept. Term 1890, Somerset County Court of Common Pleas.

141. "In a good week they generated $30...," Kimmel Nicklow, June 4, 1995.

141. "Upon discovering the mistake, Ephraim became angry...," Ibid., Oct., 31, 1991.

141. "Another time, when grandchildren complained of hunger, he retorted...," Ibid., July 22, 1989.

141. "They also grieved for son Linc, who was briefly married...," Victor Clyde Miner, interview with the author, Grantsville, Md., Oct. 26, 1989.

Part VIII - Civil War Reunions and Final Years

142. "In the 1880s, having relished two decades of peace, the nation underwent a resurgence...," Edwin C. Bearss, "Gettysburg" seminar, Western Pennsylvania Civil War Round Table, Sewickley, Pa., April 30, 1994.

143. "At an 1918 event, the *Somerset Herald* named him among 'a remarkable assemblage of aged men'...," *Somerset Herald*, Sept. 11, 1918, as reprinted in the Laurel Messenger, Feb. 2011, pp. 955-956.

144. "The outside world sometimes wonders why old soldiers love each other...," *Connellsville Courier*, Sept. 22, 1893, p. 1.

145. "When the Pennsylvania Memorial was dedicated at Gettysburg in September 1910...," "Veterans at Gettysburg," *Somerset Herald*, Sept. 28, 1910, as reprinted in *Civil War Diaries of Capt. Albert Heffley and Lt. Cyrus P. Heffley*, published by the Berlin Area Historical Society, printed by Apollo, Pa., Closson Press, 2000, n.p.

145. "While there, Martin visited his birthplace at Hexebarger but after returning home...," *Connellsville Weekly Courier*, Oct. 20, 1905.

145. "Within an hour after arriving home, said the Connellsville newspaper...," *Connellsville Daily Courier*, Oct. 2, 1915, p. 1.

146. "One of Nancy's grandsons, Donnus Franklin Farabee, recalled a visit...," Donnus F. Farabee, interview with the author, Amity, Pa., July 4, 1988.

147. "In reporting on the gathering, the Connellsville Daily Courier said Ephraim...," *Connellsville Daily Courier*, Aug. 15, 1920.

148. "Members of his Civil War Post were unable to attend the funeral...," *Somerset Herald*, March 16, 1921, p. 4.

149. "In August 1924, she and sons John and Harry and their families were among...," *Meyersdale Republican*, Aug. 14, 1924.

149. "She and her children and grandchildren went to the first event in 1926...," *Connellsville Daily Courier*, Aug. 31, 1926.

149. "The Harbaugh Reunions continue today in Farmington...," Harbaugh Reunion Archives, 1926-2000, published on Minerd.com website.

150. "He published a related newspaper, the Younkin Family News Bulletin...," Charles Arthur Younkin of Charleroi, Pa., published eight editions of the newspaper between 1937 and 1941—Christmas 1937; April 30, 1938; August 5, 1938; December 20, 1938; August 10, 1939; March 15, 1940; Sept. 25, 1940; and June 30, 1941. The newspapers were in a six-page, five-column tabloid format, at a subscriptin price of $1.00 per year. The first issue, dated Christmas 1937, was loaded with family stories and obituaries, a reunion wrapup and letters. All eight were reprinted in a booklet of the same name in 2008 by Mark A. Miner.

150. "Writing in a manuscript history of the event, Grant's cousin and reunion president Otto Roosevelt Younkin...," Otto R. Younkin, *History of the Younkin Reunion*, Masontown, Pa., 1934, republished on Minerd.com.

150. "In October 1935, Charleroi Charley traveled for an overnight visit...," Charles A. Younkin, Charleroi, Pa., letter to Otto R. Younkin, Oct. 15, 1935.

150. "She returned home safely, as Harry gratefully penned...," Harry David Miner, Markleton, Pa., diary entry, Oct. 17, 1942, (unpublished), private collection.

150. "Her double-cousin Albert "Ward" Minerd, of Mill Run, Fayette County, noted her funeral...," Albert W. Minerd, Mill Run, Pa., diary entry, Sept. 26, 1953 (unpublished), private collection.

151. "Ephraim's newspaper obituaries have been reprinted over the years...," Rockwood Historical Society, *Down the Road of Our Past*, 1995. Also see *Laurel Messenger*, Nov. 2005 and Samuel G. Miller, *A Place Called Hexie*, Bloomington, Ind.: AuthorHouse, 2010, p. 244.

151. "On July 26, 2003, a granite and bronze monument to the 142nd Pennsylvania...," *Dedication of a Monument to the 142nd Pennsylvania Volunteer Infantry*, no author, Somerset, Pa., July 26, 2003.

152. "Their mission: 'to save this land forever'...," Civil War Preservation Trust plaque, Slaughter Pen Farm, Fredericksburg, Va.

BIBLIOGRAPHY

Alcott, Louisa May. *Hospital Sketches*. Boston: James Redpath, Publisher. 1863.

American Catholic Historical Society of Philadelphia. *Records of the American Catholic Historical Society of Philadelphia*, Vol. VIII, 1897.

Barnes, Joseph K. *Medical and Surgical History of the War of the Rebellion*. Part III, Vols. I and II, prepared by Charles Smart. Washington, D.C.: United States Government Printing Office, 1888.

Bates, Samuel P. *History of Pennsylvania Volunteers 1861-1865*. Harrisburg, Pa., 1870.

Bearss, Edwin C. "Gettysburg" seminar, Western Pennsylvania Civil War Round Table, Sewickley, Pa. April 30, 1994.

Blackburn, E. Howard, William H. Welfley and William H. Koontz. *History of Bedford and Somerset Counties, Pennsylvania*, Vol. II. New York: Lewis Publishing Co., 1906.

Boyts, Hiram. *Laurel Messenger.* Historical and Genealogical Society of Somerset County, May 1989.

Catton, Bruce. *A Stillness at Appomattox*. Garden City, N.Y.: Doubleday & Company, Inc., 1953.

------. *Glory Road*. Garden City, N.Y.: Doubleday & Company, Inc., 1952.

------. *Never Call Retreat*. Garden City, N.Y.: Doubleday & Company, Inc., 1965.

------. *This Hallowed Ground*. Garden City, N.Y.: Doubleday & Company, Inc., 1956.

Berlin Area (Pa.) Historical Society. *Civil War Diaries of Capt. Albert Heffley and Lt. Cyrus P. Heffley*. Apollo, Pa.: Closson Press, 2000.

Connellsville Courier newspaper, Connellsville, Pa.: Sept. 22, 1893, Oct. 20, 1905, Oct. 2, 1915, Aug. 15, 1920, Aug. 31, 1926,

Dedication of a Monument to the 142nd Pennsylvania Volunteer Infantry,
no author, Somerset, Pa., July 26, 2003.

Downey, James W. *A Lethal Tour of Duty: A History of the 142nd Regiment
Pennsylvania Voluntary Infantry, 1862-65.* Indiana University of Pennsylvania
Graduate School Department of History, 1995.

Dyer, Frederick Henry. *Compendium of the War of the Rebellion.* New York:
Thomas Yoseloff, Publisher, 1959.

Epler, Percy Harold. *The Life of Clara Barton.* New York:
The Macmillan Company, 1915.

Farabee, Louis Thomas. *Genealogy of the Farabees in America.*
Washington, D.C.: 1918.

Foote, Shelby. *The Civil War: A Narrative. Fredericksburg to Meridian.*
New York: Random House, 1963.

------. *The Civil War: A Narrative. Red River to Appomattox.*
New York: Random House, 1974.

Forney, C.H. *History of the Churches of God in the United States of North
America.* Harrisburg, Pa.: The Publishing House of the Churches of God,
1914.

Freeman, Douglas Southall. *Lee: An Abridgement in One Volume by Richard
Harwell.* New York: Simon & Schuster Inc., 1997.

------. *Lee's Lieutenants: A Study in Command.*
New York: Charles Scribner's Sons, 1942-1944.

Gay, James D., "Satterlee U.S.A. General Hospital, West Philadelphia,"
print, courtesy of Library Company of Philadelphia.

Gearhart, Edwin C. *Reminiscences of the Civil War.* Stroudsburg, Pa.:
Daily Record Press. No date.

Goss, Rev. Charles Frederic. *Cincinnati: The Queen City, 1788-1912.*
Vol. I. Chicago and Cincinnati: The S.J. Clarke Publishing Company, 1912.

Greve, Charles Theodore, A.B., LL.B. *Centennial History of Cincinnati and
Representative Citizens,* Vol. I. Chicago: Biographical Publishing Company, 1904.

Harbaugh Reunion Archives, 1926-2000. Minerd.com.

Henderson, George Francis Robert. *The Campaign of Fredericksburg, Nov.-Dec., 1862*. London: Kegal Paul, Trench & Co., 1886.

Holliday, John Hampden. *Indianapolis and the Civil War*. Indianapolis: Edward J. Hecker, 1911.

Holloway, W.R. "Treatment of Prisoners at Camp Morton." *The Century Illustrated Monthly Magazine*, 1891.

Horwitz, Tony. *Confederates in the Attic*. New York: Vintage Books, a Division of Random House, Inc., 1998.

Howell, George R. and Jonathan Tenney. *History of the County of Albany*. New York: W.W. Munsell & Co., 1886.

Index to the Executive Documents of the House of Representatives for the Second Session of the Forty-Fourth Congress. Washington, D.C.: Government Printing Office. 1877.

Knable, Jerome B. *Diary of Corp. Jerome B. Knable*. Transcript, Historical and Genealogical Society of Somerset County, Inc.

Lee, A.E. *History of Columbus, Ohio*, Vol. II. Munsell & Co., 1892.

Leslie, Mrs. Frank. *The Civil War in the United States, 1895*.

Love, William DeLoss, Jr., Ph.D. *The Fast and Thanksgiving Days of New England*. Boston: Houghton, Mifflin and Company, 1895.

Meyersdale Republican newspaper, Meyersdale, Pa.: July 17, 1913, Aug. 14, 1924

Miller, Samuel G. *A Place Called Hexie*. Bloomington, Ind: AuthorPress, 2010.

Miner, Edward John. Conversation with the author, Washington, Pa. Oct. 29, 1978.

Miner, Harry David. Private diary, Markleton, Pa., unpublished, private collection.

Miner, Mark Alan. Minerd.com biographies of Leroy Bush, Thomas C. Custer, Michael A. Firestone, Henry "Foxy" McKnight, Mary "Hester" (McKnight) Strauch, Adaline (Harbaugh) Minerd, Albert Miner, Alpheus Minerd, Andrew Jackson Miner (of Ohio), Catherine (Miner) Bedillion, Charles Minerd, Daniel L. Minor, Eli Minerd, Elias Minor, Elizabeth (Miner) Lindley, Ephraim Miner, Frederick Miner Jr., Henry Minerd, Henry Harrison Minerd, Hester (Minerd) Rankin, Jemima (Minerd) Burditt, Joanna (Minerd) Enos, John Minerd, Laveria (Minerd) Georgia, Martha Emma "Matt" (Minerd) Gorsuch, Martin Miner, Nancy (Minor) Farabee, Rebecca (Minerd) Behme Kearns, Rosetta (Harbaugh) Miner, Samuel Miner (of Ohio), Sarah (Minerd) Shepard, Susan (Miner) Birch, Susan (Minerd) Rose, Susanna (Minerd) Mayle Woody, Leonard Rowan, Eli Van Horn, Isaac Van Horn (www.minerd.com).

------. "Family Is Everything." *Pittsburgh Quarterly*. Fall 2008.

Minerd, Albert Ward. Private diary, Mill Run, Pa., unpublished, private collection.

National Park Service. *Fredericksburg and Spotsylvania County Battlefields.* U.S. Department of the Interior. No date.

New York Herald. Dec. 18, 1862.

O'Reilly, Francis Augustín. *The Fredericksburg Campaign: Winter War on the Rappahannock.* Baton Rouge: Louisiana State University Press, 2003.

Pitman, Benn, ed. *The Assassination of President Lincoln and the Trial of the Conspirators.* Cincinnati: Moore, Wilstach & Baldwin, 1865.

Rable, George C. *Fredericksburg! Fredericksburg!* Chapel Hill: University of North Carolina Press, 2002.

Randall, J.G. and David Herbert Donald. *The Civil War and Reconstruction,* 2nd Ed. Lexington, Mass.: D.C. Heath and Company, 1969.

Reid, Whitelaw. *Ohio in the War: Her Statesmen, Generals and Soldiers,* Vol. I. Cincinnati: The Robert Clarke Company, 1895.

Reports of Committees of the Senate of the United States, for the Third Session of the Thirty Seventh Congress. Washington, D.C.: Government Printing Office, 1863.

Rockwood Historical Historical & Genealogical Society, *Down the Road of Our Past,* 1995.

Sandburg, Carl. *Abraham Lincoln: The War Years, Vol. I.* New York: Harcourt, Brace & World, Inc., 1939.

Somerset County Leader. "Ephraim Miner." March 1921.

Somerset Herald. "Mrs. Ephraim Weimer," March 31, 1875. "Veterans at Gettysburg," Sept. 28, 1910. "Remarkable Assemblage of Aged Men." Sept. 11, 1918; reprinted in the *Laurel Messenger,* Somerset, PA: Historical and Genealogical Society of Somerset County, Vol. 51, No. 1, February 2011. "Ephraim Miner," March 1921.

Studer, Jacob Henry. *Columbus, Ohio: Its History, Resources, and Progress.* 1873.

Terrell, W.H.H. *Indiana in the War of the Rebellion.* Indianapolis, Douglass & Conner, 1869.

United States Census, 1860. Somerset County, Pa., and Marshall County, Va.

United States Christian Commission for the Army and Navy. *First Annual Report.* Philadelphia: 1863.

------ for the Year 1864. *Third Annual Report,* Philadelphia, April 1865.

------. *Third Report of the Committee of Maryland.* Baltimore: James Young, 1864.

United States Pension Files. Washington, D.C., National Archives Building: Michael A. Firestone Application #117033, Certificate #79017, Widow App. #1143973, Cert. #879930. Jacob Pritts App. #163879, Cert. #114822. Simon Pile App. #189254, Cert. #128484, Widow App. #615916, Widow Cert. #418846. David Gohn App. #76552, Cert. #47225. Frederick F. Iams App. #104267, Cert. #101962, Widow App. #848818, Widow Cert. #618371. Chance Minor App. #451291, Cert. #495033, Widow App. #1000614, Widow Cert. #756377. Adam Nickelson App. #320854, Cert. #470448. Cyrenus W. Newcomb App. #765852, Cert. #692403. Wesley Long App. #786397, Cert. #583993, Widow App. #591719, Widow Cert. #405337. Nelson Oscar Sharp App. #599618, Cert. #750560, Widow App. #1133435, Widow Cert. #874722. Chauncey Brockway App. #998279, Cert. #876838. George F. Rollins App. #558048, Cert. #385738, Widow App. #420379,

Widow Cert. #325364. Daniel Ash App. #93751, Cert. #65931, Widow App. #371658, Widow Cert. #249817. Sylvester DeMary App. #95863, Cert. #68911, Widow App. #946297, Widow Cert. #710967). Amos Hartdorn App. #211141, Cert. #142871. Leonard Grose, App. #105504, Cert. #102464, Widow App. #1072385, Widow Cert. #818758, Minor App. #1015968, Minor Cert. #795566. Frederick Brauhn App. #274082, Cert. #171266, Widow App. #302325, Widow Cert. #200392. David Kifer App. #822405, Cert. #609374, Widow App. #842160, Widow Cert. #636180, XC #2678251. Ephraim Minor App. #308962, Cert #264987, Widow App. #1172852, Widow Cert. #903476, XC 2703889 (lost). Chance Minor, App. #451291, Cert. #495033, Widow App. #1000614, Widow Cert. #756377.

Walkinshaw, Thomas. *Local and National Poets of America, with Interesting Biographical Sketches from Over 1000 Living American Poets.* Chicago: American Publisher's Association, 1890.

Warren, Horatio Nelson. *Two Reunions of the 142d Regiment, Pa. Vols.,* also known as *War History,* Buffalo, N.Y.: The Courier Company, 1890.

Whitman, Walt. *Complete Prose Works.* Philadelphia: David McKay, Publisher, 1892.

------. Letter to Louisa Van Velsor Whitman, May 25, 1865. Courtesy of the Walt Whitman Archive (www.whitmanarchive.org).

Younkin, Charles Arthur. Letter to Otto Roosevelt Younkin. Charleroi, Pa.: Oct. 15, 1935.

Younkin, Otto Roosevelt. *History of the Younkin Reunion,* Masontown, Pa., 1934, republished on Minerd.com.

ACKNOWLEDGEMENTS

I wish to thank several good friends who kindly reviewed this manuscript and made excellent suggestions for much-needed improvements. They include cousin Sharon (Sheldon) Kern of Findlay, Ohio and her husband, Dr. G. Richard Kern, a national authority on the history of the Churches of God; cousin Melody Gary of Beaver Falls, Pennsylvania; and Francis Augustín O'Reilly, author of *The Fredericksburg Campaign: Winter War on the Rappahannock*, and National Park Service historian at the Fredericksburg battlefield.

Above all, I wish to acknowledge my parents, O. Wayne and Constance Miner, for cultivating a love of family, books and history, and to my patient wife Liz for enduring the peculiarities of married life with a writer.

Ephraim Miner's broad story is scattered among many libraries, archives and research facilities. All of them have contributed to this work in some way, and I am grateful for their excellent resources and service.

Ancestry.com
Beaver Area Memorial Library, Beaver, Pennsylvania
Berlin Area Historical Society, Berlin, Pennsylvania
Biesecker Memorial Library, Somerset, Pennsylvania
Bowlby Public Library, Waynesburg, Pennsylvania
Brooklyn Public Library, Brooklyn, New York
Carnegie Free Library of Connellsville, Pennsylvania
Carnegie Library of Pittsburgh, Pennsylvania
Churches of God Historical Society, Findlay, Ohio
Citizens Public Library, Washington, Pennsylvania
Cornerstone Genealogical Society, Waynesburg, Pennsylvania
Fredericksburg National Battle Park, Virginia
Google Books
Library Company of Philadelphia, Pennsylvania
Library of Congress, Washington, D.C.
Meyersdale Public Library, Meyersdale, Pennsylvania
National Archives, Washington, D.C.
National Park Service, Fredericksburg, Virginia
Northland Public Library, Pittsburgh, Pennsylvania
Rockwood Historical Society, Rockwood, Pennsylvania
Senator John Heinz Regional History Center, Pittsburgh, Pennsylvania
Uniontown Public Library, Uniontown, Pennsylvania

ABOUT THE AUTHOR

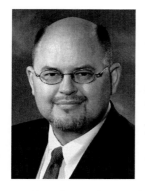

Mark A. Miner is an award-winning writer, editor and publisher who has had a lifelong interest in the Civil War. With a journalism degree from West Virginia University, he has built a career spanning more than a quarter of a century, and in 2005 was named to the Renaissance Hall of Fame of the prestigious Public Relations Society of America for his contributions in the fields of law, engineering and accounting. Since 2002, he has been CEO of Mark Miner Communications, LLC (www.markminer. com), a corporate communications consultancy serving professional service firms, and in 2011 he established Minerd.com Publishing, LLC. He is active in board leadership roles with the American Cancer Society in Pittsburgh and Beaver (PA) Area Heritage Foundation and Museum. Since 1995, he has served as president of the national Minerd-Minard-Miner-Minor Reunion, and since 2000 has been webmaster of Minerd.com (www.minerd.com), named by Family Tree Magazine *as one of the top 10 family websites in the nation. He and his wife Liz reside in Beaver, Pennsylvania, a suburb of Pittsburgh.*

INDEX

Minerd, Alpheus: 97, 160
Minerd, Charles: 122-123, 161
Minerd (Miner), Eli: 125
Minerd, Grant: 122
Minerd, Henry: 18, 20-22, 117, 121, 161
Minerd, Jacob Sr.: 13
Minerd, Jacob III: 20
Minerd, James Jr.: 78
Minerd, Joanna Younkin: 89, 123, 134-135
Minerd, John: 20, 52
Minerd, Josephine (see Hall, Josephine
    Minerd)
Minerd, Lawson: 122, 161
Minerd, Lucinda J. (see Hall, Lucinda J.
    Minerd)
Minerd, Martha Emma (See Gorsuch,
    Martha Minerd)
Minerd, Maria Nein: 13
Minerd, Polly Younkin: 18, 20, 116, 154
Minerd, Rebecca (see Kearns,Rebecca
    Minerd Behme)
Minerd, Rebecca "Jennie" (see Woodmency,
    Rebecca "Jennie" Minerd Conley)
Minerd, Sadie (see Luckey, Sadie Minerd)
Minerd, Sarah Ansell: 52
Minerd.com Website: 14, 146, 149, 152, 154,
    158-159
Minor, Chance: 20, 22, 66, 77, 88, 116, 159
Minor, Daniel L.: 64, 158
Minor, Elias "Eli": 116, 125, 161
Minor, Elizabeth (see Armstrong, Elizabeth
    Minor Wilson)
Monocacy Junction, Maryland: 71, 159
Monroe, James: 27
Mount Pleasant U.S. General Hospital,
    Washington, D.C.: 131
Mud March: 44, 52,
Mulcahy, Nellie: 124

Narragansett, R. I.: 63
Nassau, N.Y.: 128
National Archives, Washington, D.C.: 13, 36,
    55, 130-131, 154, 156-162
National Day of Fasting and Prayer: 113
National Park Service: 152, 171
Navy Yard, Washington, D.C.: 56-57
Never Call Retreat: 67-68, 158
New Hampshire Infantry Regiments: 13th:
    129
New Jersey City (see Jersey City)
New Jersey Infantry Regiments: 8th: 130
New York City, N.Y.: 16-17, 80-81
New York Artillery Regiments: 2nd (Heavy):
    130. 7th: 129. 9th (Heavy): 130

New York Infantry Regiments: 2nd: 126.
    22nd (National Guard): 129. 116th: 127.
    121st: 129. 169th: 126-128
Newark, N.J.: 130, 161
Newcomb, Cyrenus W.: 126-127
Newport News, Va.: 126, 129,
Nickelson, Adam and family: 63, 158
Nickler, William: 36
Normalville, Pa.: 117, 144-145
North Anna River, Va.: 65-66
Northrup, E.W.: 128

O'Reilly, Francis Augustín: 28, 34, 156, 171
O'Laughlin, Michael: 59
Oblong, Ill.: 150
Ohio Cavalry: 10th: 64
Ohio in the War: 112
Ohio Soldiers Home: 111
Ohio Volunteer Infantry: 19th: 59, 84, 158.
    34th: 98. 90th: 77, 159. 122nd: 127. 144th:
    71, 78
Ohiopyle, Pa.: 147-148
Ohler, Alice Pearl (see Miner, Alice Pearl
    Ohler):
Old Bethel Church of God: 19-21, 122, 135,
    141, 154,
Old Town, Maine: 131
Orange Turnpike, Va.: 64
Orcutt, Peter V.: 127
Our American Cousin: 106

Paddytown, Pa.: 18, 134
Peeble's Farm, Va.: 84
Pennsylvania Artillery Regiments: 5th: 136
Pennsylvania Reserve Regiments: 3rd, 4th,
    7th, 8th: 33, 36
Pennsylvania Cavalry Regiments: 16th: 117
Pennsylvania Infantry Regiments: 62nd: 132.
    85th: 78, 159. 140th: 55, 93. 142nd: 23-40,
    44-48, 52, 54, 63-69, 75, 78-80, 84, 87, 91,
    99, 102-103, 105, 111-112, 142-144, 151,
    156, 158, 164. 155th: 75. 188th: 89.
Pennsylvania Memorial, Gettysburg: 145
Petersburg, Va.: 15, 55, 68-69, 75-76, 78, 80,
    84, 88, 93, 99, 103, 129, 158,
Pettit, Isabelle Farabee: 122, 124, 161
Pettit, William: 122
Philadelphia, Pa.: 16-17, 45-49, 80-81, 120,
    131, 156-157, 159,
Pickett, George E.: 103
Pickett's Charge: 42
Pierson Tract, Fredericksburg, Va.: 33
Pike's Peak, Colo.: 138

United States Christian Commission: 91, 93, 157, 159-160
United States Constitution: 98
United States House of Representatives: 98
United States Postal Service: 135
Ursina, Pa.: 149-150
Utica, N. Y.: 120

Van Dyke, Louiten: 55
Van Horn, Eli: 71, 159
Van Horn, Isaac: 78, 159
Veterans Administration: 13, 162
Veterans Reserve Corps (VRC): 48, 55. *22nd*: 82, 85, 87, 97, 123, 126-131
Vicksburg, Miss.: 131, 142
Vining Station, Ga.: 77

Walgren, Doug: 13
Walter, H.: 124
Walter Reed Army Hospital: 72-73
War History: 54, 143, 154, 158, 160
Warner, Horace B.: 129
Warren, Horatio Nelson: 24-25, 28, 54, 64-66, 68, 76, 91, 99, 102-103, 105, 143-144, 154-156, 158-160
Warrenton, Va.: 25
Warrington Junction, Va.: 128
Washington, D.C.: 16, 24, 27, 45-46, 48, 55-56, 65, 73, 80, 95, 101, 106-107, 111, 128, 145,
Washington, George: 27
Washington, Mary: 27
Waynesburg, Pa.: 117, 146-147, 171
West Middletown, Md.: 119
Wheeling, W. Va.: 129
Weimer, David: 36
Weldon Railroad, Va.: 78-79, 84, 91
West Fort Ann, N. Y.: 127
West Virginia Cavalry Regiment: 1st: 66
West Virginia Infantry Regiment: 10th: 129
Western Maryland Railroad: 149
Whipkey Family: 135-137, 149
White House, Washington, D.C.: 74, 107,
White House Landing, Va.: 126, 128
Whitman, George: 41
Whitman, Walt: 17, 41-42, 46, 49, 55-56. 58, 65, 74, 111, 156-160
Wilderness Battle: 15, 63-64, 67, 130
Williams, Pa.: 146
Wilson, Woodrow: 145
Winchester, Va.: 129
Windmill Point, Va.: 44, 46

Woodmency, Rebecca "Jennie" Minerd Conley: 122, 161
Woody, Fleming: 99
Woody, Susanna Minerd: 99
World War I: 147

Younkin, Charles Arthur ("Charleroi Charley"): 149-150
Younkin, Ephraim: 18
Younkin, Freeman: 135
Younkin, Harmond (Herman): 121, 134, 161
Younkin, John F.: 121
Younkin, John J. "Yankee John": 20-21, 106, 134,
Younkin, Otto Roosevelt: 150, 154, 163
Younkin, Polly Hartzell: 134
Younkin, Susan Faidley: 134
Younkin Cemetery: 134-135
Younkin Family News Bulletin: 150, 163
Younkin, Lucinda Harbaugh (see Johnson, Lucinda Harbaugh Younkin)
Younkin National Home-Coming Reunion: 150

Zanesville, Ohio: 116
Zufall, Aaron: 44-45, 157